ONE STEP OVER THE LINE

ONE STEP OVER THE LINE

A No-Nonsense Guide to Recognizing and Treating Cocaine Dependency

Joanne Baum, Ph.D.

1817

Harper & Row, Publishers, San Francisco

Cambridge, Hagerstown, New York, Philadelphia,
London, Mexico City, São Paulo, Singapore, Sydney

ONE STEP OVER THE LINE: *A No-nonsense Guide to Recognizing and Treating Cocaine Dependency.* Copyright © 1985 by Joanne Baum, Ph.D. All rights reserved. Printed in the United States of America. No part of this book may be used or reproduced in any manner whatsoever without written permission except in the case of brief quotations embodied in critical articles and reviews. For information address Harper & Row, Publishers, Inc., 10 East 53rd Street, New York, NY 10022. Published simultaneously in Canada by Fitzhenry & Whiteside, Limited, Toronto.

FIRST EDITION

Library of Congress Cataloging-in-Publication Data

Baum, Joanne.
   One step over the line.

   Bibliography: p.
   1. Cocaine habit.   2. Cocaine habit—Treatment.
I. Title.
HV5810.B38   1985   362.2′93   85-42769
ISBN 0-06-250045-7

85 86 87 88 89   RRD   10 9 8 7 6 5 4 3 2 1

Dedicated to the people I have worked with and those who may benefit from this book

Contents

Acknowledgments

I would like to thank Sapir Weiss, who first suggested that I write a book about cocaine. He and his wife, Jane, both good friends, had been listening to me talk about my work for a year and a half. One evening he said, "Why don't you write a book about what you do with these people who are having trouble with cocaine?" Around the same time, I gave a paper ("Treating Cocaine Abuse: The Upside and the Downside") at the San Francisco Chapter of the Society for Clinical Social Workers. It was very well received, and the members suggested I expand it into a book. These people continued to be an important support, asking about my progress each month. They had faith from the beginning, when I was still wondering if this idea would become a reality.

I could not have written this book without the people I have worked with. Without them—their work, their lives, and their sharing—this book would not have been possible. I have learned from them just as they have learned from me and our work together.

I also want to thank the Haight Ashbury Free Medical Clinic Detoxification Project, and in particular Dr. David Smith and Darryl Inaba, Ph.D., who provided me with an incredible work experience. I am still amazed at how much I learned in the two years I worked there. They launched my career in chemical dependency treatment.

I would also like to thank some people who have contributed their professional advice and supportive friendship throughout the writing of this book: Gil Weisman, M.D.; Millicent Buxton; Carole Campana, Ph.D.; Michael Berlin, Ph.D.; Maureen Bush; Bill Henkin; and Dorothy Gibson. My parents, Bill and Elaine Baum, have never failed in their weekly or biweekly phone calls to ask how the book is going. Michele Driscoll has edited my writing chapter by chapter, teaching me things I never learned in school; and Christine Schlemm has typed the manuscript with all its notes, inserts, and changes. They have all been excited about the project and encouraging all along the way.

I also want to acknowledge some people I have known in a more personal way, whose drug problems made me think, take a step back, and wish I could do something for them. I haven't been able to help them directly, but maybe this book will help them get past some of their own denial, which up until now has blocked them from getting any help. They know who they are. To you people who helped introduce me to the seductive and insidious qualities of cocaine, I thank you.

My husband and co-therapist, Timothy M. McCarthy, helped me to keep my perspective as I was writing this book. Tim's knowledge and experience in the chemical dependency field has greatly influenced my work. He was willing to talk over ideas; and at times he suggested that I not talk over ideas, that I leave the book alone and let it go. Both these roles were very much needed at different times. He has also been a wonderful co-therapist for groups, families, and couples—it is a pleasure working with him.

Judy Coburn, a free-lance writer and friend, edited the first prospectus I wrote and helped get me going. The National Writers Union, San Francisco Chapter, gave me invaluable information on publishing and provided me with a recommendation for a lawyer, Brad Bunnin. As it turned out, Brad was the one who suggested that I send my manuscript to Harper & Row.

I want to thank Clayton Carlson and Matt Chanoff at Harper & Row for their initial interest in the book and for their continued excitement and support. I am sure there are other people who helped make this time so pleasant. I enjoyed writing, and on some days only wished there were more hours in the day so I could write more.

Introduction

BY DAVID E. SMITH, M.D.

Due in great part to such pioneering treatment professionals as the author of this book, we have learned a great deal about the nature and treatment of cocaine abuse. What is being learned is alarming, but it is leading us steadily toward more effective treatment of what is obviously a growing problem.

In the 1960s and through most of the 1970s, cocaine was not considered dangerous. Due to complex and interrelated social, cultural, and pharmacological influences, cocaine was thought of by consumers and health professionals as a relatively benign drug. Many felt that insufflation (**snorting**[1]), the most common means of using cocaine, was self-regulating because of the drug's vaso-constrictive qualities. Consequently, cocaine use could not result in addiction, overdose, toxic psychosis, or death.

Our experience at the Haight Ashbury Free Medical Clinic, however, led us to different conclusions. In the late 1960s we witnessed what could only be called an epidemic of amphetamine abuse. Methamphetamine (**speed**), a central nervous system stimulant similar in action and effect to cocaine, had also been considered a "safe" drug.

These fears were confirmed as the late 1970s brought a significant increase in cocaine abuse, overdose deaths, and acute toxicity involving physical, psychological, and behavioral dysfunction. Between 1980 and 1983, first-time admissions of cocaine abusers had increased to 19 percent of all first-time admissions to our clinic. Increases throughout San Francisco were similarly significant. From 1978 to 1983, the death rate from cocaine overdose in

---

1. Drug-related terms set in bold-face type are defined in Appendix A.

San Francisco went up 300 percent. Los Angeles, Denver, Miami, and other urban centers had similar reports on abuse and overdose deaths. Once more, we are facing a stimulant epidemic.

This epidemic has gone beyond what are considered to be recognized drug-abusing populations. Nearly 75 percent of the new cocaine abusers are employed. As a group, they tend to be "treatment naive"—they have not had repeated contact with the drug treatment system. They are not traditional drug abusers or addicts aware of programs that might be available to help them.

Most importantly, they are victims of the myth that cocaine is a safe, benign, and non-addicting drug. Their awareness of cocaine's hazards came only after they became users, and the myth, coupled with their own denial, often keeps them from treatment until the situation has become exacerbated.

Cocaine withdrawal is not subject to the life-threatening seizures that can complicate alcohol and other sedative-hypnotic withdrawal, nor does it involve the physical symptomatology of opiate analgesic withdrawal; thus cocaine is often considered non-addictive. This view is totally in error. Our treatment of more than three thousand outpatient cocaine abusers has shown that cocaine addiction—characterized by compulsion, loss of control, and continued use despite adverse consequences—is a major outcome of abuse. Thus cocaine addiction fits very closely into the disease model of addiction.

Joanne Baum has a broad base of clinical experience in working with chemically dependent clients and their families. Her work with a wide variety of abusers from the drug culture while working at the Haight Ashbury Free Medical Clinic, coupled with her experience as a private practitioner, gives this excellent book a diverse foundation leading to a sensible and effective approach to the treatment of cocaine abuse and addiction.

Preface

In some ways I felt compelled to write this book. At a time when cocaine has a reputation as a fun and harmless drug, people in unprecedented numbers are checking themselves into chemical dependency treatment programs for problems with cocaine. Cocaine has caught us all off guard. The media has given so much attention to the cocaine hype—the glitter, the Hollywood scene, the musical scene, the so-called fun of the drug—that I felt a need to balance these images with the unromantic reality.

In my private practice as a therapist specializing in chemical dependency treatment, I have seen many clients who dangerously abuse or are addicted to cocaine. This book is based on my work. The situations you will read about reflect what I have actually encountered. Some of the characters may look familiar to you because many addicts have similar stories, though the people I discuss are fictitious, often composites of several people. The work that I do has changed over the last few years, and I assume this will continue as I learn from my patients. The stories and treatment strategies contained in this book reflect the current state of the art in the chemical dependency field.

I have written this book for many people: therapists, concerned family and friends, and for cocaine users. I sometimes get phone calls from colleagues who don't know what to do with patients who are using too much cocaine. Treating chemical dependency is not an easy task. They have heard about my work and want to know what I am doing. I also hear from people who are worried about family members and friends. They call to ask how much cocaine is "too much," and what they should do with a spouse or friend they suspect is abusing cocaine. Cocaine addicts themselves often want to be treated differently than alcoholics and other drug addicts. They claim they have "special problems." Do they? Most cocaine addicts I have seen initially come in for treatment of what they describe as a cocaine "problem," and want to know how they can use cocaine recreationally again; they want to get control of their drug usage. It's hard for them to believe that once they have abused a drug to the point of addiction, they can never "get control of it" again.

Cocaine gets people into situations they never thought they would be in. For instance, yelling at your kids or colleagues or crying at your desk is not "fun," but it is what people have done when they are at their wits end after a cocaine **run** and have lost perspective on the world around them. Being paranoid and hiding in closets so "they" don't find you after you've just snorted up a gram of cocaine isn't "fun," but many people have found themselves crouched in a corner, hiding. Gripping the bathtub with a needle stuck in your arm, trying not to pass out and hit your head on the cold tile floor, is not exactly "fun" either—but it is something people experience while they are still looking for that old elusive **high**. These kinds of feelings and experiences are real. I have heard about them, in varying forms, many times.

Addiction is a family disease. It is very powerful. In tight groups of friends, and in some instances family groups, people can actually support each others' denial of drug problems. They become more emotionally and physically drained as time passes, while insisting they are having "fun." Denial can go so deep that even in the face of death a supportive group can say (and believe) the person died of "respiratory failure"—even though that respiratory failure may have been cocaine induced, and the person may have had no previous medical history of respiratory problems. Somehow, people are able to maintain their distorted perspective of reality.

This book is written for those people, and for others who may be a little more open to recognizing the consequences of drug use, drug abuse, and drug addiction. I hope that if you are wondering about yourself or about someone else, you will read on.

This book is also written for professionals in the mental health,

health, and chemical dependency fields who are baffled by patients who use cocaine and other drugs. I particularly want to share with you some of the methods used in recovery programs and the reasons why these methods can work.

When I first began to work at the Haight Ashbury Free Medical Clinic Detoxification Project, a "success" was defined as a person who had stayed clean for one year, or even as a person who had cut down a habit. As I worked more closely with Dr. David Smith, I learned about a treatment process based on an idea called the "disease model," which suggests addiction is a disease that can only be treated with abstinence from all drugs and a life-long recovery program. I also began to see more and more value for recovering addicts in **Alcoholics Anonymous**, **Narcotics Anonymous**, and **Cocaine Anonymous**. These programs, with their **twelve steps**[2] for recovery, have been most successful in maintaining the sobriety of millions of people. Initially, the notion of AA did not sit well with me—I had some of the same blocks I was later to encounter from my clients: "All that God stuff, forget it." But if it might benefit the people I was working with, I was willing to give it a try. I went to a few meetings, talked to people who had been working with the disease model for years, and talked to people who had been living the program for years. When a couple of my clients slipped— began to use cocaine again—I decided to try incorporating this model into my therapy. And it has worked. Abusers and addicts need to change their entire lifestyle if they are going to be able to stop using drugs and live a healthy, full life. They are going to need new supports and new resources. We work on this as part of their recovery program.

Cocaine is no respecter of gender. In my practice I see a fair mixture of men and women, although the balance seems to shift from time to time. Cocaine is also not limited to a particular group of people. Since it is so widespread among all social classes and throughout the country, it is very likely that you know

---

2. See Appendix B for the twelve steps and twelve traditions.

someone involved with cocaine; if so, this book may be a real eye-opener for you. You may be surprised to see your boss, your friend, your partner, or even yourself on these pages. Perhaps not all of it will "fit" you, but, "take what you liked and leave the rest."[3]

3. *This Is Al-Anon*, copyright 1981, by Al-Anon Family Group Headquarters, Inc. Reprinted by permission of Al-Anon Family Group Headquarters, Inc.

1. What's All This Fuss About Cocaine?

Each day, five thousand people try cocaine for the first time. I see them at the other end of the trial, when cocaine has become an overwhelmingly powerful and destructive force in their lives. They can't handle it alone; they need help. The men and women I work with come from diverse backgrounds, but they all have one thing in common: a drug problem. Each one has suffered psychologically, financially, and often physically from doing too much of what began as a "good" thing, a "fun" thing.

How much cocaine is "too much"? Too much is when you start using it even when you know you've had enough. Too much is when you start feeling fearful, paranoid, irritable, nervous, enraged or panicky. Too much is when your heart starts racing uncontrollably. Too much is when your nasal membrane starts getting eaten away. Too much is when all your money goes to buy cocaine. Too much is when you decide to stop doing cocaine, but find yourself buying it anyway. Too much is when cocaine becomes more and more important in your life. Too much cocaine may be a gram a week, half a gram a day, two grams a day, four grams a day, or even six grams a day; it varies from person to person.

People seek my help for a variety of reasons. Some are frightened and nervous, either because they have begun to feel one of the negative consequences of doing too much cocaine—uncontrollable paranoia—or because they are just scared to face the reality that they need help. Most are simply sick and tired of feeling sick and tired. The common thread that binds them all together is the realization that drugs have been playing too significant, or too negative, a role in their lives. They may not know that they are addicted, or that they have a problem; but they know something is very wrong. And at least part of them wants to find out what that something is and get rid of it, so they can get on with their lives unhampered by the mysterious problem.

No matter how much resistance a person first presents to therapy, I always give them credit for coming in. Something made them come to my office. Something inside them wants to face the problem, and facing a problem head-on is the first step to dealing with denial, the tall wall that separates a person in trouble from a person in recovery.

"AM I USING TOO MUCH?"

Here's an example. I received a phone call from a young woman who was worried that she might have a drug problem. She said she wasn't sure, but would be interested in talking to me and seeing what I thought. I agreed to meet with her.

"Barbara" was a waitress in a well-known restaurant, recently arrived from Milwaukee, and not quite used to the lifestyle she found in San Francisco. She said she was constantly exposed to cocaine at the restaurant; customers as well as fellow workers offered it to her at least four times a night. At first she had stayed clear of the drug, but after about two months of constant contact she occasionally said "yes" to the offers. By the time she came to see me, not only was she saying "yes" to all offers, but she had begun to buy half a gram almost every day. "I know half a gram isn't all that much, but on my salary I'm beginning to feel a real crunch. My rent is late for the first time . . . I can pay it if I just don't buy any coke for a couple of days. I wonder about my drug use, but in comparison to people around me, mine is nothing, so maybe I'm okay."

I asked Barbara if she thought the cocaine was affecting her in any other way besides the obvious financial burden. She said, "No, I don't think so, I'm really not using *that* much." I asked her if she noticed any mood swings. "What do you mean?" she retorted rather defensively. "I mean, are you more moody than usual? Do you have more highs and lows than you're used to?" She looked at me with her head cocked to one side. "Well, now that you mention it, I guess I have noticed myself being a little more on edge. Does that mean something?"

"Let's talk some more before we come to any hasty decisions here. At this point I'm just trying to gather information so I can best tell you what I think is happening, and then I want to tell you a little about cocaine. Then we can decide what to do. Okay?" "Yeah," she said. "I guess I just got a little scared."

I assured her that it was natural to be scared, this was scary stuff we were looking at. I told her it showed a lot of willingness and health on her part to call for help as soon as she realized the increasingly significant role cocaine was playing in her life, instead of waiting until her life had become unmanageable.

Some people, like Barbara, are lucky. They come in for help as soon as they realize that their cocaine use has gotten out of hand. Others are not so lucky. They wait until they have lost their jobs, their homes, their families, their cars, everything they had worked so hard for.

One young man who called me talked very fast and frenetically on the phone. "Hello, I got referred to you by . . . by . . . actually, I've been making so many phone calls today I don't even know who referred you, but I got your name and whoever it was said you were real good and might help me. Will you?" I told him that I needed a little more information before I would know if I could help him or not. "Look," he said, "I'm not feeling too well, and I need to know if you can help me." I asked him what he needed help with, and he proceeded to launch into a long monologue.

Well, I guess it's me. I'm just so self-destructive, always have been, you know, the black sheep in the family and all. It's hard, it's real hard right now. Even though I was the black sheep I managed to get my own business going, my very own, and I was even staying afloat, making it happen— me, the black sheep. Then I guess I went and did what I always do, but it was different this time. I messed it up. It was my own self-destructiveness at work. I destroyed my business. I mean it's still there, they haven't kicked me out of my store yet, but I'm barely hanging on. I lost my apartment, I'm sleeping in the back room at my store. I had to sell my stereo and most of my furniture to pay rent here and, I guess some of it went to the **blow**. A lot of it went to the blow. And my girlfriend. She even left me when she saw my business going down the tubes. She didn't want to be with a nobody. As long as I was making money she was there, but when I started on my self-destruct path she split. I want to stop doing this stuff, but I can't seem to. I even got some more coke this morning and did it instead of going in to see the loan officer at the bank, and I have to do that. I have to straighten up some financial matters if I have any intention of keeping this business. I don't want to mess up all the good things in my life, but I do. Can you help?

After this man and I had worked together, he came to discover that he was not a self-destructive person. Rather, he learned that he had a disease—cocaine addiction—which had caused his life to be totally out of control and unmanageable. After he had been drug free for a while, he also came to the conclusion that his girlfriend had probably left him because his behavior was very erratic and upsetting to her, not because he was running out of money. He had physically threatened her several times in an attempt to make her get him more coke at times when he wanted more, but was incapable of leaving the apartment to get it for himself. Following his threats, she had gotten up in the middle of the night, left the apartment, and bought him some coke. He came to see that that was too much to ask, that she didn't want to be a part of his disease, and had left to take care of herself since she couldn't help him. He also admitted that he had sold a few of her things along with his to buy drugs, and had lied to her about it. He began to see that he had built up a large wall of denial, and had hidden behind it to avoid taking responsibility for his behavior. He blamed others, he blamed his so-called self-destructiveness, he blamed anything but the real culprit: cocaine.

Fortunately, he was able to salvage his business. Months later, he was even able to talk to his old girlfriend, apologize for his behavior, and tell her about his recovery. She greeted the news with mixed feelings; her trust was not what it had once been. He said he felt guilty that she was still hurting so badly, but observed,

Once I would have used my guilt as an excuse to go out and use coke, but now I know I don't have to do that. It's a relief. I can feel sadness, and even pain now, and not run away from it. I know it'll pass, and I'll feel a lot better a lot sooner if I stay away from drugs. That instant relief I used to look for really doesn't last. Instead, I would end up feeling worse than I had before. Sometimes it's amazing to me how much I denied for so long, but most of the time I understand it, especially when I remember I have a disease that makes it real easy for me to deny and distort reality.

He was beginning to live one day at a time, getting through each day without doing drugs, staying away from his old haunts and his old friends. He knew he needed a new lifestyle if he was going to beat the image of being "nothing but a self-destructive brat in a man's body," which is the way he had once described himself to me. He was also able to talk to his family about his addiction, and to get some new-found respect from them. He began by telling them on his own, and later he brought them in for some family work, where we were able to deal with it more therapeutically.

Even though his cocaine habit was much more expensive than Barbara's, in many ways their recovery was similar. Both crossed over the line into addiction from simple recreational drug use or drug abuse, and both had to stop using cocaine and all other drugs.

Barbara had left our first session armed with information about cocaine. She was determined to prove that she had caught herself in time. She thought she could stop using cocaine, because she now knew it was a highly addictive drug and she didn't want to become addicted. Unfortunately, she had already become addicted. She had been so sure she could pay her rent "just a few days late; I just won't buy any coke till its paid. The landlord said I could have a few days."

Three weeks later, faced with eviction, she called me again. It hadn't been that easy to stop using cocaine. In fact, she found it was an hourly struggle that was getting to be too great for her. She said, "In order for me not to use, I have to tell myself over and over again that I shouldn't. And even then it just means that I don't do as much as I want—I haven't stopped using. I mean to say 'no' at work and instead I say 'yes.' I think I'd better come in again. I don't want to, but I don't think I have much choice right now."

When she came in she told me about other things that had been happening in her life. Some of them had started before she saw me for the first time, but at that point she had not been willing or able to attribute them to the cocaine. She was currently on probation at work, because she had been arriving late and getting edgy with customers. One night, about an hour after she had finished her day's supply of coke (the amount she was going to allow herself), she had actually started yelling at a customer who wanted to change his order for the third time. Her justification at the time was, "He was just stoned and didn't know what the hell he wanted. Why should I have to take that crap?"

In retrospect, she realized that if she hadn't been coming down from cocaine herself she probably would have laughed at his behavior. Her roommate had also been complaining about her "inconsiderate" behavior, her odd hours, and her sleeplessness and prowling around the house all night. At the time she had blamed her sleeplessness on the move, on going through a tough transition; but she forgot that before she had started doing cocaine, when the move was even fresher, she had slept fine.

It took her a few weeks to tell me that during the last month of her usage, around the time she had first called me, she had started drinking regularly. She had never thought of herself as a drinker; so even though her alcohol consumption had increased drastically (right along with her cocaine consumption), she didn't pay any attention to it. Her denial was simple: She never had been a drinker, and therefore she still wasn't. Denial is an incredibly strong mechanism in addiction. It allows a person to keep using and keep doing things long after common sense has said, "Let's stop, I think I've had enough."

"WHAT HAPPENED TO MY WILLPOWER?"

Many people come into my office and say, "I don't understand, I want to stop." Or, "This is crazy. I'm unhappy, I feel lousy, I want to stop using cocaine, but I keep doing it anyway. What happened to my willpower?"

Addiction has nothing to do with willpower. I have worked with many people who have a lot of willpower, they are very strong-willed and stubborn people. The disease of addiction is stronger than they are, it's stronger than all of them put together. It's only when addicts begin to feel better, begin to not use—when they admit that they are powerless over the drug and cannot control their usage—that the fierce battle can end and recovery can begin. It may seem inconsistant, but it's true. My co-therapist, Tim McCarthy, has said, "An addict cannot *not* use. What comes naturally to an addict is using drugs."

Addiction is a chronic, often relapsable disease; despite this, I have seen people turn their lives around. I have seen people give up drugs and learn to have fun in different ways. Some people, however, are not so fortunate; and they have contributed to a 600 percent increase in cocaine-related deaths between 1970 and 1980. We can assume that this has continued to increase in the 1980s, because so much more cocaine is being smuggled into this country each year.

At least 5,000 people try cocaine for the first time every day. It is unclear how many people use cocaine regularly, but estimates range from 15 million to 25 million. Cocaine use among young professionals in their twenties and thirties seems to be doubling every year.[1] Given these figures, and the fact that cocaine can kill, the picture soon becomes frightening.

Cocaine is the world's most highly psychologically addictive drug. The National Institute on Drug Abuse (NIDA) suggests that 20 percent of people currently using cocaine will become addicted. Most people using cocaine do not even know it's addictive, don't believe it's addictive, or believe they are part of the

---

1. Statistics are from the National Institute on Drug Abuse.

safe 80 percent. Unfortunately, you usually don't find out that you're part of the 20 percent until you are addicted, and then there's no going back to recreational drug usage of any kind. Going back would be playing a dangerous game of Russian roulette with your life.

Cocaine is so highly addictive, in fact, that it usually takes people by surprise, especially people who have considered themselves immune to drug problems. Just because you have managed to drink socially for fifteen years does not prove that you are beyond addiction. Many people I see professionally have worked very hard for a long time to get where they are, in their personal lives and in their jobs. They have paid their dues and are beginning to reap the benefits. They feel they deserve a break, that it's about time they relaxed a little and had some fun.

Cocaine provides these people with a great respite from their routine. Initially, it is a quick high that guarantees a lot of fun in a short period of time. So they go for it. But those who go for it in a big way often find the fun is replaced by other, less pleasant feelings, which are often ignored until they become overwhelming. The negative feelings that have replaced the fun feelings seem to last longer, but somehow people find reasons to continue using cocaine long after the fun is gone. Where is that quick, once certain, now elusive high? Where did it go? Some people chase it down blind alleys, running into all kinds of brick walls along the way, burrowing under, slamming through, climbing over, all in a more and more frenetic search for more cocaine, more fun, and more relief.

One of the most insidious characteristics and symptoms of addiction is that people try like hell *not* to get better; their denial of the problem overrides their common sense. They are not in control of their lives, but they are unaware of that fact. It is only when they reach the end of their rope that I see them. When they do come for help, they are once again looking for relief. They want to feel better, and they are very anxious to feel better quickly. After all, they are important people with a lot of things to do and people to see.

Usually, new patients don't think cocaine is the culprit. They may think it's part of the problem, but it is not usually the identified problem. So what's all the fuss about? Maybe it's only a symptom of something deeper.

"IS COCAINE THE CULPRIT?"

People like myself who work with cocaine addicts are continually amazed at the range of powerful problems that result from overuse of the drug. Nervousness, irritability, anger, rage, paranoia, discomfort, anxiety, and depression are all feelings addicts experience. They are often financially and emotionally bankrupt, and they are completely out of touch with what was once important to them. Marriage, children, work, and self—all fade in comparison to the all-important, all-consuming need to acquire and use cocaine.

One woman, "Linda," called me because she was worried about her husband's behavior.

Linda: I don't understand what has happened to my husband, Jed. He's acting so strangely; it's like Dr. Jekyl and Mr. Hyde moved in and my husband moved out. We've always been so compatible, but now . . . I'm truly worried. I don't know if it's his job, or me, or something he's not telling me. I've even wondered if it's another woman. I would be almost relieved to know it's another women—at least we could deal with that. He's so irritable, yelling at the drop of a hat, trouble sleeping . . . things that used to make him happy just don't anymore. It's making me so upset.

I'm five months pregnant and I had felt so good about having this baby till all this started. We waited— I'm thirty-six and my husband is thirty-eight—we had wanted to provide the child with a stable home environment, and we could have, but now . . . I just don't know. We both have very good jobs. But the stress or something is getting to him. But why now? Maybe having the baby is stressing him?

I've tried talking to him, but he won't even talk anymore. Sometimes it's the way it was, and he'll bring home flowers or a nice bottle of wine, but other times it's like I don't even exist. He seems interested in something else and he'll stay in his study for hours. I'm just at my wit's end. I don't know what to do.

Therapist: What does he do when he's closeted in his study?

Linda: I'm not sure. Sometimes he locks the door. I guess he reads, or daydreams, or works, or, or . . . now that I'm thinking about it, I have found small squares of shiny magazine paper in the garbage; they look like the packets that cocaine sometimes comes in. There's also a mirror and a razor in his top drawer. I'm reluctant to even say this because I've never looked in his things before. We are both rather private people and respect that in each other, but it's been getting so bad. He leaves the house at all hours of the night. And comes back to his study.

Therapist: Do you have any idea what your husband might be doing?

Linda: The only thing I'm talking about that I haven't really looked at as a possibility is the cocaine. I'm not too knowledgeable on the subject. We both smoked marijuana in our day, but less and less frequently through the years. Neither one of us comes from a home where there was much alcohol—socially, of course, but our parents are strictly social drinkers. We enjoy having wine with dinner, but not to excess. Neither one of us has ever had a drug problem of any kind. In fact, when we started trying to get pregnant I gave up all drinking and drugs. It was not a problem at all, it was something I wanted to do.

We were only introduced to cocaine last year. My husband had met some people at his new job, and they always seemed to have it along. It seemed that we both could either take it or leave it, but when it was offered we felt it was the socially gracious thing to accept. But we never bought any. No, that's not true. My husband had arranged to have a gram at a party we gave about six months ago, so we could reciprocate. I've never looked at this before. It is true that we had agreed we would both stop the drinking and the little drug use we had been doing when we started trying to get pregnant, although now that I think of it, I stopped but he didn't. I really never thought about it before.

As it turned out, this couple had worked very hard every since leaving college to make a successful life for themselves. Linda was an accountant with a large, successful firm, and Jed was a lawyer who had started in the public defender's office and after two years moved into a small corporate law firm. He had remained in that firm until the last year, when he had been hired by a large and prestigious company. That's when cocaine was introduced into their lives.

After several phone calls and a few cancelled sessions, we were able to bring the husband in for counseling. Initially, Jed was reluctant to see any connection between what he called a "temporary adjustment problem" and his cocaine use. It was only when his wife was able to bring hard, cold evidence of the changes in his life that he was able to admit a possible connection. She had to show him the books, his budget, and explain what a mess they were in financially, before he was willing to budge from his firm stand. Then she confronted him with his mood and behavior patterns. He was finally able to see how appealing cocaine had become for him.

Jed: It was great. I have always been a private person, but, after snorting some cocaine, I was gregarious and carefree without having to work hard at it. I liked that. Also, I have a tendency to overbook myself, so I don't have a lot of time to relax. Cocaine helped there, too. It was like when I first smoked marijuana in the '60's, I would feel an almost instant sense of relaxation and peace. Cocaine was like that. I would feel a sense of contentment with myself at first, but it was a more animated comfort that allowed me to be social. And when my wife stopped doing any drugs because we were trying to have a baby—well, I know I had agreed to go along with her, but I was having too much fun. And she didn't push the issue. Somewhere in there I can see it got out of hand. But don't you think, after all these years of handling drugs, that I can handle this one too?"

Therapist: It depends on what you mean by handling it. If you mean that you want to cut down on your cocaine consumption, I think, from what we've learned about your usage, you'll have trouble. If you mean you can begin a recovery program and handle that, that's a different story. You seem like a person who is interested in feeling better now that you are beginning to face the reality of what your life has become. It must have been pretty lonely sitting in your study, by yourself, locking your wife out of your life, and snorting cocaine all through the night.

Jed: I'm not sure I'm convinced yet, but I can see how important cocaine has become. It's true, I did lock my wife out of my life, and she has always been very important to me. No wonder she thought I might have a mistress. I did, only her name was cocaine. I couldn't have had sex with another woman if I had wanted to. I seem to have lost interest in that too, somewhere along the line.

I and a co-therapist worked with this couple together, and also saw each spouse separately; the husband on a regular basis, the wife periodically. They were each able to begin a recovery program of their own and find new ways of communicating with each other. It wasn't easy, but it was possible. By the time their baby was born, they were both completely drug free and had been for a few months. We will talk more about how people recognize their problems and how treatment works in later chapters.

WHAT DO YOU BELIEVE?

Here's another fairly common situation. "Carolyn," a young woman, admitted that she had a cocaine problem, and was willing to abstain from cocaine. But she was initially unwilling to abstain from other drugs or even see how other drugs had become a problem. During our early sessions she was trying to control and dictate her recovery program. She said she would abstain from drugs, but that alcohol really wasn't a problem and she "chose" to continue to drink. I will work with people in this situation for a relatively brief period of time, hoping they become more willing to give up control and listen to another point of view about their situation. During our third session I confronted her.

Therapist: This is a scenario that works well for a lot of people. I'd like you to tell me what you think about it. Once people have **copped** and used coke, they often try to feel better as they are coming down, to cut the **edge** off. Well, people usually do that with a less stimulating drug, like Valium or alcohol.

When people repeat this pattern of getting high and coming down, they often inadvertantly develop what we call a "cross" or "secondary addiction," becoming addicted to more than one drug. And although they may be more willing to see cocaine as a problem—after all, it's depleting their financial resources or making them do things they had never considered doing (resorting to extortion or embezzlement to get money for their drug)—they often don't see their secondary drug usage as a problem. After all, it was used for "medicinal" reasons, to come down more easily, to ease the crash, to help them feel better. But whatever the reasons for its use, the other drug has also become a problem; it too is part of the addiction process. Sometimes it's hard for them to reconcile that not only has their drug of choice gotten out of hand, but perhaps another drug has too. How does that fit with you?

She had become visibly uncomfortable as I was speaking—squirming around in her chair, playing with her hair, looking at the floor. She was having trouble looking at me. There was silence before she responded, and then she spoke in a low tone, her voice shaking with emotion.

Carolyn: I see myself in there, but I swear it was like you say. I saw my drinking as a way to feel better—like if you had bad cramps with your period, you drank some brandy. I never recognized the connection. I guess I did wake up with hangovers. I just attributed that to lack of sleep. I guess I have a lot to think about . . .

This book will probably give you a lot to think about too. It presents my experiences with cocaine abusers and addicts over the last few years and offers a model for treatment that has been successful. From what I have seen, I believe that people who have become addicted—who have become compulsive in their drug use, lost control of that use, and continue to use in the face of negative effects—must abstain from *all* drug use. No more alcohol, no more marijuana, no more sleeping pills when they're anxious and can't fall asleep, no more recreational use of drugs. Even prescription drugs (in particular, any mood-altering drugs) must be used with caution and be prescribed only when absolutely necessary and with the person's addiction in mind.

Most drugs that we traditionally see as addictive are physiologically addictive. Cocaine is psychologically addictive, but the process of addiction, the process of the disease, and its debilitating and chronic nature are the same. So, although a person's symptoms may look like emotional problems, or even be as severe as a psychotic break, treatment by traditional psychotherapy or psychoanalysis will not "cure" the drug addiction.

In addition to the psychological addiction, cocaine can cause physiological problems: irregular heartbeats, high blood pressure, sudden drops in blood pressure, nasal and sinus problems, respiratory difficulties, perforated nasal cavities, paralysis, and heart attacks. It is entirely possible to die from relatively small doses of cocaine, especially if one is already prone to seizures, high blood pressure, or heart or respiratory problems.

Users should also be concerned about substances that might have been added to the cocaine to increase its weight, and therefore its market value. Substances that have been used to **cut** the cocaine can cause serious physical damage and even death. For instance, lidocaine, a substance frequently used to "step on" (cut) cocaine, can cause respiratory paralysis and the inability to breath. Lidocaine taken in too large a quantity will cause death from suffocation. What is too much? We don't know—and if you bought some coke that had been cut with lidocaine, you wouldn't know either. Since you couldn't find out how much was in it, you wouldn't even be able to know if the coke you had purchased had "too much."

HOW TO USE THIS BOOK

If you are a family member or friend of someone who enjoys cocaine, what should you do? Unfortunately, there are no pat answers. This book will supply you with the necessary information to help you see if the person you care about is having a problem with cocaine, if he or she has become addicted, and if so, what options you have. It will also give you information about the drug and its effects, which you can pass along to the user. Or you can encourage the user to read the book. More important, you will be able to make informed decisions about what you want to do with this unexpected intruder—cocaine—in your life.

Addiction is a family disease, and its effects inevitably spill over to everyone around the user. Everyone around the addict tries desperately to make sense out of the craziness that ensues with addiction. Let me assure you: It can get less crazy, recovery programs can work, and life can be less painful and more fun.

Therapists and medical professionals who are baffled by those patients who won't get better will find some clues in this book. Addicts do not really engage in traditional transferential rebellious behavior, rather, they exhibit symptoms of an active disease. I am frequently amazed that after a person is in recovery, and has been clean of all drugs for a while, many of the previously seen symptoms of uncooperative and rebellious behavior disappear. The therapist is often surprised at the change. Only after a person has been drug free for a period of time, and has learned about the disease and what it will take to stay drug free, can more traditional issues be explored. The haze of active addiction no longer distorts all messages going in and out, though even during this phase of treatment the therapist or physician needs to be aware of the part addiction still plays in a drug-free addict's life. A person in recovery will still exhibit patterns of the disease, such as obsessive behavior and a strong desire to have everything happen now. These issues are all dealt with in a recovery program.

If you are a cocaine user, take a look at this information. It is not readily available on the streets, but you ought to consider it when you are thinking about using. You may not have crossed over the line into addiction, but even if you have, there are alternatives. You just need the willingness to act as if there could be something different for you. Remember: Since you may have a disease, you can get some help if you are thinking about abstaining from drugs. You don't need to do it alone.

In the next chapter we'll look at cocaine use through history. One philosopher said, "If we do not learn from history, then we are doomed to repeat its mistakes." So let's look back at where all this came from before we assess where we are now and where we could go from here.

2. Cocaine the Seductress

Cocaine has been popular during three different periods of history: during the Incan Empire in South America (A.D. 800–1000); from the late 1890s to about 1906; and, in our own time, it has enjoyed a steady rise in popularity since the mid-1970s. In fact, it never has been as popular as it is today. The stimulus that seems to trigger cocaine's availability to the general public is different each time, yet the same themes—a reputation for being mystical, powerful, and seductive—seem to prevail. Today a new theme has been added: having fun.

Cocaine is the new social drug. Word has it that if you have cocaine you'll have fun, you'll be able to pick someone up, you'll be able to party and have a good time, and sex will be much better. People will respect you if you have cocaine. The more you have and the better it is, the more of a following you'll have.

How have these popular myths surrounding cocaine arisen? Why is cocaine seen with such reverance? A look at cocaine's history will help establish a precedent for the phenomenon we are seeing and experiencing today.

THE INCAN EMPIRE: ECONOMIC INCENTIVE

During the period A.D. 800–1000 the Incan Empire considered coca leaves (from which modern-day cocaine is made) as a godlike substance. It was treated with the utmost reverence and respect. Coca leaves were used in religious rituals and by holy men in order to improve their memory so they could orally transmit the sacred myths; they also felt it improved their ability to prophesy. Cocaine was used by nobility during religious services and during special festivities, and it was also sometimes provided to non-nobility as a reward for a particularly heroic deed.

According to myth the first coca plant grew from the earth in which an Incan Queen was buried. This was not just any Incan Queen—she had been accused of being an adultress and summarily killed. Thus coca's connotation as a seducer is ancient.

After the Spanish arrived in South America, the use of coca leaves spread very quickly. The conquerors discovered that the coca leaves had anti-fatigue qualities, reduced the appetite, and made people less sensitive to temperature changes. They encouraged the Indians to chew coca leaves while they worked. As a result, their endurance was greatly increased; they could work longer and harder and produce larger profits for the Spanish rulers. Unfortunately, the Spanish rulers ignored the fact that a worker's body was eventually going to need to catch up on that sleep, food, and rest that had been neglected while the leaves were being chewed. When those deficits were not made up, the result was a shortened life span; Indians only lived to be about thirty years old.

THE LATE-NINETEENTH AND EARLY-TWENTIETH CENTURIES: MEDICAL INCENTIVE

Alfred Niemann isolated the principle alkaloid from coca leaves, and was able to transform them into a purified substance that became known as cocaine. Shortly after this discovery, pharmaceutical companies began to market cocaine and send it to physicians for use in various medical contexts.

Perhaps the best-known and most detailed account of this early phenomenon was documented by a relatively unknown physician, an ambitious man looking to make his mark in medicine—Sigmund Freud. One of Freud's ambitions was romantic. In love with a woman from a wealthy family, he had to prove himself to her family by achieving fame and fortune in order to be granted her hand in marriage; he saw cocaine as the answer to his dreams. After early use and experimentation with the drug, Freud called it a panacea and documented its curative powers in alleviating many ailments, including melancholia, nervousness, and addiction to morphine and alcohol. In the late 1880s Freud went to the World Conference of Physicians in Vienna, hoping to receive notoriety for his recently published work on the values of cocaine. Instead, he was blamed for introducing the world to "the third scourge of addiction" (the other two being morphine and alcohol). Freud left the conference dejected and abandoned his research with cocaine. It was only years later that his book, *Uber Coca*, was discovered under the floorboards of his home.

During the time when Freud was gaining and then losing the respect of the formal medical community, the rest of the world was off and running in its support of cocaine as a panacea. Patent drug companies sold numerous medicines that included cocaine as the main ingredient; various elixirs made with cocaine were being sold door to door or from the general stores housed in wagons and carts that roamed the countryside in the United States.

During this second phase of popularity, massive doses of cocaine were prescribed for tuberculosis victims. One of the people so treated was none other than Robert Louis Stevenson, who, under the influence of the drug, wrote the book *Dr. Jekyll and Mr. Hyde* in just a few days. It is no coincidence that today I often treat people who say that they feel like Dr. Jekyll and Mr. Hyde, because they can't control their emotional responses, that they think they may be developing a split personality or going crazy. This syndrome, today known as **cocaine psychosis**, was first metaphorically documented in Stevenson's popular book.

Another popular figure of the times, the fictional character Sherlock Holmes, reflected his creator's relationship with cocaine. Arthur Conan Doyle, author of the Sherlock Holmes detective stories, was a cocaine addict who used the drug to combat the severe depressions with which he struggled throughout his life. In fact, Conan Doyle is credited with discovering the euphoric qualities of speedballing—injecting a mixture of cocaine and morphine—hence the line, "Quick, Watson, the needle!"

During the 1890s—when cocaine was being accepted by the general public as a wonder drug, and was being openly used by some notable and romantic characters of the time—the formal medical community was beginning to question the efficacy of using cocaine in medicines that were sold without a prescription. Its addictive qualities were being documented more frequently and were beginning to alarm the medical community. The following report by a Dr. Baudry reflects the feelings of the medical community at the time: "The most alarming poisonous effects of the drug are: debasing and enslavement of the will, a general demoralization which is as diabolical as it is indescribable, and which tends rapidly toward depravity and to the development of everything that is degrading and ignoble in human nature."[1]

At the same time that these reports were filtering through to the public, a new soft drink was introduced. Asa Candler bought the formula for Coca Cola in 1891 from a pharmacist, John Pemberton, who had originally marketed it as a prescription drug to be used for headaches, hysteria, and melancholia. When Candler bought the formula he transformed it into a soft drink flavored with coca leaves and the kola nut, and braced by a small amount of cocaine. Coca Cola could be purchased at soda fountains, and was widely advertised as a tonic and restorative. (The cocaine was removed from Coca Cola in 1904; but by then Coca Cola's popularity was established and the company still profited, despite the absence of its addictive ingredient.)

In 1906 the Pure Food and Drug Laws were passed. They succeeded in eliminating cocaine and opium from drugstore shelves, except in some medicines that were regulated by prescription and supposedly were monitored to prevent abuse.

Following the medical community's reticence to use cocaine, and the subsequent legislative response, cocaine fell from popularity. It was hardly ever seen or talked about (except within two small subcultures: artists and musicians, and a small group of criminal figures) until the 1970s.

---

1. Quoted by Sidney Cohen, *Cocaine Today* (New York: The American Council on Marijuana and Other Psychoactive Drugs, 1981), p.15.

FROM THE MID-1970s TO TODAY: HAVING "FUN"

For seventy years cocaine was hardly used. What happened during the 1970s to make cocaine so popular again? Stories of fun times and wild parties began creeping out of the Hollywood scene, out of the musicians' carefully guarded subculture, and into the popular press. Cocaine began to be thought of as the drug that a connoisseur would enjoy, just as one would enjoy a find bottle of champagne—to be indulged if one could afford it. Cocaine became the symbol of having "made it." It conferred such a desirable status that more and more middle- and working-class people began to think of cocaine as something to have on special occasions. Because of its addictive qualities, some people found that "special occasions" began to occur more and more frequently.

Within the last ten to fifteen years, frequency of cocaine use has risen enormously. The cocaine trade is an industry now ranked somewhere between Ford Motor Company and Standard Oil of Ohio. Its associated sales of related paraphernalia has been con-servatively estimated in value at an annual $30 billion and grow-ing (Gold, 1984). In 1982 approximately 45 to 54 metric tons of cocaine had been smuggled into the United States; federal offi-cials estimate that close to double the amount was brought in during 1983. Viewed as a fun drug and a harmless drug by a naive public, cocaine has taken and continues to take an appalling toll of human life and happiness every year (San Francisco Sunday Examiner and Chronicle, 1984). Between 1977 and 1980, cocaine-related deaths increased 600 percent; and that figure is still rising. Admissions to drug programs for cocaine have also risen mark-edly in the last five years (Seidler, 1982).

Confronted with these facts, many people simply deny their significance. "Look," they say, "plenty of people I know do cocaine and they're doing fine." Because they don't want to believe that cocaine is a dangerous drug, many people continue to deny it all the way—until they are broken financially, emotion-ally, and physically. Ironically, denial itself is symptomatic of addiction and allows the disease to perpetuate itself.

One of the most seductive qualities of the drug has contributed to its recent rapid rise in popularity: its initial positive effect. Cocaine has the ability to create certain euphoric feelings. Initially, it makes people feel powerful, on top of the world, in control, confident, and happy—at least for a while. But cocaine also has the opposite effect. It can create an extreme dysphoric state, producing depression, paranoia, and psychotic behavior. This reality of cocaine, however, is not widely acknowledged.

Cocaine is seductive. It lures a person in with its initial positive effects, then produces more and more negative effects which are not noticed at first, because thinking is distorted by the cocaine. Eventually, as the user tries time and again to get **high**, to recreate the initial positive feelings, cocaine takes control. The person is no longer controlling the usage, but rather responding to an involuntary craving for the drug.

It is important that the information known about cocaine a hundred years ago again becomes common knowledge. Only in this way can people make an informed decision when cocaine is offered to them, a decision based in reality.

3. King of the Mountain

Cocaine use has spread like wildfire since the 1970s. On February 19, 1984, an Associated Press news story from Washington began, "Despite a multi-million dollar campaign against narcotics, the United States was inundated last year by a wave of smuggled cocaine, and federal drug enforcers are digging in for a long battle . . . (San Francisco Sunday *Examiner and Chronicle*, 1984). Why is this battle going on today? What are the powers of this drug? What is its lure? How does cocaine attract its users?

I've talked to many people about their history with cocaine, and I always ask, "Why did you start? What made you start using?" The reasons I have been given fall into six groups: (1) "It's got such a mystical aura and reputation, I was just curious"; (2) "It was available and being offered"; (3) "It made me feel good about myself, it gave me a sense of well-being"; (4) "It made me feel accepted by a group"; (5) "It was a great way to escape"; and (6) "It was a way to sabotage my success and flirt with 'the edge.' "

Perhaps for all of these reasons, cocaine currently enjoys an elevated social status as the "in drug" to have and to be using. Most newcomers to the cocaine scene do not know cocaine is addictive; and even if they have heard that tidbit of information, they are quite sure they are not susceptible to addiction. These people are all afflicted with what I call **white powder blindness**, the "it won't get me" syndrome. This chapter examines the reasons people start to use cocaine, and then looks at the paradoxical consequences of these initial positive motivators.

"THE MYSTICAL REPUTATION AROUSED MY CURIOSITY":

Curiosity about cocaine is a major reason some people begin using the drug. The myth of cocaine's origin from the burial place of an adultress queen of the Incan Empire carries a mystical and sexual hype that still lives today. An additional part of cocaine's mystique today derives from its identification with the elite. A number of my clients from lower-and lower-middle-class backgrounds have said it made them feel important; knowing they were doing what the elite were doing gave their ego a boost. If they could not mix with the elite directly, socially or professionally, at least they could mix with them indirectly by sharing their lifestyle. Upper-class people say their friends talked about it so much and were doing it so much that it aroused their curiosity; what began as idle curiosity developed into a major habit and lifestyle. One woman said, "Cocaine became so prevalent in my life that instead of getting a cup of coffee for a quick pick-me-up, I'd just sit down and have a couple of lines. I could justify it by the amount of time I saved."

A huge industry has arisen around cocaine paraphernalia, increasing the drug's already ritualistic aspects. People can chop their cocaine on special marble slabs, glass frames, or mirrors; these objects are usually reserved for the sole purpose of getting the coke ready to be **snorted**. Such items as knives, credit cards, razor blades, and even gold razor blades are used to chop the cocaine. The drug is then inhaled through everything from a rolled dollar bill—or a hundred-dollar bill; to a plastic, brass, or gold straw; or even a tiny spoon—again, made from anything from brass to gold. (I recently saw a man in a bar proudly pull out a shiny-new brass straw he had just received and pass it around among his friends, who oohed and aahed as it passed from hand to hand. Then someone said, "This calls for a celebration," and pulled out a small packet of shiny magazine paper, unfolded it, and began laying out **lines** on the bottom of a glass ashtray. The new straw was then "christened" by the Birthday Man.)

People who **freebase** have their own elaborate rituals to get the cocaine ready. It must be dissolved in water, an alkali added, then the pure cocaine is extracted using a flammable solvent. The cocaine is then smoked in a pipe. Freebasers go through larger quantities of cocaine than snorters, because during the process of purifying the cocaine by getting out all the cuts they lose about three-quarters of the substance and are left with the pure cocaine portion (which on the streets is about 20 to 25 percent of the purchased amount). That will go very quickly in a pipe, so people generally buy more at a time or keep returning to their dealer for more. If a snorter went through the same quantities of coke as a freebaser, the membrane between the nostrils would soon be perforated.

Shooting cocaine involves an entirely different ritual. As one man who used coke **IV** said:

All I had to do was see my **rig** in my drawer and I'd get excited. I'd take it out, play with it a while, and the next thing I knew I'd be at the dealer's house. I hardly remembered how I got there, I was just there, and then I was home **fixing** it—putting it in the needle and then shooting it in my arm. I really liked pulling back on the needle and getting just a little bit of blood in the syringe, knowing I had hit the vein and was about to shoot that coke in and straight for my brain. What a **rush**! I tell you, I felt great, just great, until I came down. Then I wanted more, or if my wife came in, I'd feel guilty, real guilty.

More recently, the mystical aura surrounding cocaine has been joined and thereby heightened by a sexual hype (one of its street names is "the white bitch"). Shooting drugs has had sexual connotations for years: "I put the needle in her arm, slowly pulling back on the rig, and then I shot the stuff in, slowly and evenly . . . I sat back and watched her face light up and knew she was feeling good . . . she was feeling real good." This imagery can certainly conjure up sexual activity. Orgasmic pleasure is simulated by the drug as it is absorbed by the veins and quickly, within seconds, hits the brain and then the person's whole body with a temporary state of euphoria. As one man said, "We bask in the white bitch's powers."

Cocaine is said to enhance sexuality, prolonging and heightening sexual excitement and increasing orgasmic feelings. This may be true for recreational and occasional users; but high doses of cocaine can actually reduce sexual activity and impair a man's ejaculatory and erectile abilities. Again, these facts are not commonly talked about among cocaine abusers and addicts; so when users experience sexual impotence they get worried, scared, and feel inadequate, which worsens the problem. Often, until they come for treatment, they treat their feelings of inadequacy with a self-medicating prescription—more cocaine—which, instead of alleviating the problem, exacerbates it. A number of people have entered treatment with impotence as a problem they very much want to talk about, but are too embarrassed to bring up themselves. For this reason, I often mention sexual dysfunction as a negative effect of cocaine most people don't know about, thus allowing the person to discuss it more easily. The usual reaction to my statement is, "I didn't know that, do you think that's why I haven't been able to get into it with my girlfriend so much?" We take it from there.

It seems clear that the mystical aura and the sexual hype surrounding cocaine are just that, an aura and a hype and not anything based in reality. Unfortunately, the myths are so alluring that they raise people's curiosity and they begin to dabble with it. Some people do just dabble with cocaine occasionally but for many the initial "high" and good times are so alluring that they get into a good deal of trouble with the drug. Unfortunately newcomers don't know that the high is transient and addicts don't want to give up their old images.

"IT'S AVAILABLE AND BEING OFFERED ALL THE TIME"

In my present clinical work, I have been told that a big reason why people begin to use cocaine is that it's around them and being discussed all the time. Between hearing about it and being offered it, their curiosity is raised and one day they say "yes" when it's offered. Many have said they didn't even think about their response; one day "yes" just came out. As one woman said, "Give anyone in this city a half hour, tops, and they can get a quarter- or a half-gram of cocaine. Give anyone a few hours and they can come up with a pound."

Cocaine seems to be available to men and women in all walks of life. I have worked with lawyers, accountants, cabdrivers, musicians, managers, secretaries, security guards, bus drivers, bartenders, janitors, store clerks, waitresses, architects, court reporters, stockbrokers, business consultants, advertising agency personnel, mechanics, computer programmers and analysts, factory workers, clerical workers, and hairdressers; and they all have said, "Everyone around me uses," or "It's around me all the time," or "My colleagues and my clients are always offering it to me."

Some people have told me that they had heard cocaine could be addictive, but they believed this couldn't be true when all the prestigious people they came into contact with talked about using it. Surely these people would have it more together? Unfortunately, not all the time. As one man said,

Hey, I had only snorted the stuff for a long time, you know, on and off . . . nothin' heavy, then I went to this party, and there were all these people there: judges, lawyers, doctors, and they were all doing it so I thought, "This must not be so bad." So I took a hit on the **pipe**. It seems I just couldn't stop. I lost everything . . . my house, my car, my family, and now my job. I'm on the streets, sleeping at the Salvation Army, standing in line for a meal. I'm thirty-eight years old and I've never been unemployed before . . . I gotta stop, but I'm not sure if I can . . . I may have to die first.

Because many people see friends and coworkers talking about and doing cocaine, they begin believing it to be all right, believing they are only having fun. Cocaine use has been likened to marijuana use in the 1960s; but unlike marijuana, cocaine's addictive qualities are very subtle and insidious. Not only do users become addicted, they encourage others to use as well, many of whom may also become addicted to the drug.

One client who had been **clean** for two weeks said,

Okay, so I told my three dealers not to sell me any, but so far this week three other people at work have offered me some at four different times. I didn't even know they used. I've said no so far, but hey, it's not so easy. I gotta tell them to stop offering because I can't always be expected to be so strong.

This woman worked at a low-level job in a major corporation and was complaining because she couldn't seem to get away from cocaine; it was everywhere and offered to her constantly. She no longer wanted to be part of the drug subculture, but others didn't want her to leave. They didn't really believe her when she told them that she didn't want to use anymore. Offers came less frequently when she told them she had a serious problem with cocaine and couldn't use it anymore. Even so, she reported that every once in a while people tested her, saying, "Oh, come on, you haven't used for a few months, surely a couple of lines isn't going to hurt." Little did they know just how much a couple of lines could hurt. When a person has been clean for a period of time and then starts using again, the drug usage usually escalates rapidly, becoming worse than it was before. Deaths have occurred during a first **run** following a long period of abstinence.

Today in America cocaine is available to virtually anyone. It is also true that cocaine can be turned down (it won't jump up and bite you for not partaking), and it is also true that there are people to have fun with and do business with who don't use cocaine. It only looks to the active user as though everyone is using cocaine. This is another example of white powder blindness, complicated by pressure from a cocaine-using group that supports continued use. Though sometimes this pressure can change to support for being clean, other times new friends must be found who will support an addict's recovery.

Availability is a two-edged sword. It not only heightens a person's curiosity and desire to try cocaine, availability also makes it more difficult to quit. I have seen people use cocaine's prevalence and availability as excuses to put off entering a recovery program—"I just can't seem to get away from it." Once a person is ready to stop, however, cocaine's availability isn't a factor; rather, it becomes just another reality to contend with and learn to live with, to be avoided when possible and turned down firmly when offered.

"IT GAVE ME A SENSE OF WELL-BEING, LIKE I WAS WORTH SOMETHING"

One of the qualities of a **cocaine high** is that, initially, it makes you feel powerful and in control. Of course, this feeling is short-lived (lasting two to forty minutes, depending upon the method of ingestion and the quality of the cocaine), and the crash back to reality can be rather harsh; but abusers and addicts largely ignore all negative aspects and keep going for that increasingly illusory sense of well-being.

Oh it just makes you feel so good . . . like you can accomplish whatever you want. Remember as a little kid playing "king of the mountain," racing up a hill and keeping the other kids off the top? Well, with cocaine you get that feeling of being on top of the world. It's great.

Some cocaine users say cocaine made them feel better about themselves and gave them the courage to socialize. Before using cocaine they had felt inadequate and been painfully shy; but now they believed that they could snort a few lines, go to a party, and have a good time. As one cab driver said,

You know, it's hard driving a cab for hours each day in the city, dealing with different people all the time, never knowing what to expect. And I've always been real shy, especially with strangers. Somehow I never thought what I said was important, I guess I didn't think anyone would listen. Why should they? That's why cocaine was so good for me at first. I could snort a few lines and I'd be talking like crazy. Not in a bad sense . . . I felt like I was really communicating with my passengers, I was sure I had something to say, and that felt good for a change.

Later, this same cab driver admitted that at some point the drug had taken control of him. He had begun to spend all his money, lie to his wife, feel edgy and nervous, and was beginning to get paranoid that "they" would find out or that he would **blow-it**. Even though he wanted to stop doing cocaine, he found himself obsessively thinking about it and unable to concentrate on his work. His solution had been to give in to his obsessive thoughts and **cop** some cocaine.

Cocaine can make you feel better, it can make you feel good, it can make you feel powerful and in control of your world— until it gets control of you; then cocaine acts like a sadistic seducer. As one man said, "But it hurts so good . . . and I keep waiting for her [cocaine] to be sweet again, to lift my spirits, to treat me good, but she's turned on me." It is the initial cocaine high that novices are after; and that attraction is alluring long after it fades from reality as even a remote possibility.

The flip side of the coin for the cab driver, and other people who initially like cocaine because it gets them past their shyness, is that as they use cocaine excessively and become addicted, they begin to have very different reactions. They become edgy, paranoid, sullen, and introspective. By this time other people make them nervous, and ultimately they've actually lost ground socially; they're worse off than ever. When you see someone on this flip side of feeling good, it's hard to keep in mind that their original intent in using cocaine had been to have fun.

"IT FELT GOOD TO BE A PART OF A GROUP"

A number of people I have worked with said that cocaine had initially made them feel better about themselves, and they found a group of people that they had felt comfortable hanging out with. This in turn made them feel, for the first time, a part of and accepted by a group of people. One said, "Hey, when I had cocaine I always had friends around. It was so much fun being part of all that activity and excitement."

Cocaine users tend to divide themselves into three distinct subgroups: snorters, freebasers, and IV users. People who snort cocaine hang around with other people who snort; whereas freebasers hang around with other freebasers, and have condescending attitudes towards people who snort cocaine. One man said, "I can turn down a line easily, that doesn't do anything for me. But let someone offer me a pipe and whoa, there are no stops. I won't stop till I'm broke and then I'll get my dealer to **front** me some." People who shoot cocaine intravenously have an emotional attachment to and intrigue with the needle itself, and with the act of shooting the drug into their own or someone else's veins. Some people "just love" the needle, while others won't go near one.

It is interesting to observe how cocaine is treated at parties. One woman said,

At the first party I went to with people from my new job, I was somewhat aware that the host was taking some people aside to what looked like a storage room. I didn't want to appear too nosy, but it got my curiosity. Once, when I was walking past the door, I looked inside and saw a small, low table with a mirrored top. There were lines of white powder set out. I was pretty naive at the time, having only used cocaine a couple of times, but I recognized what that was.

I didn't get invited into the room that night . . . I felt a little left out, but also a little superior because I didn't need that stuff to have a good time. It seemed like there was an in-group at this place and they were the ones escorted to the mirrored table.

I wondered what all the fuss was about; later I found out . . . A few months later I knew I was accepted when, at the next party, someone took me into the back room and there was this table with these giant lines already laid out and a brass straw, just sitting there beckoning me. . . .

It felt good to be accepted and have something in common with other people who I worked with.

One person in a recovery group said, as other members nodded in agreement,

In high school I didn't quite fit in. I wasn't friendly with the straight crowd, although I was smart, and the greasers were not my type. So I got involved and accepted by the druggies. It was nice being someone, although I wondered about it at first. Then I was too high to care.

Doubts or self-consciousness were hidden when I was high; I only felt them when I came down, so I tried to stay high as much as I could.

The group members talked about how they had the camaraderie they so desperately wanted when they found other people who liked to get high. One person said, "It felt so good and important to be important to people other than my family, because they had to accept me—they were stuck with me. But strangers. . . . " During this same group discussion a member said, "I got so that I knew if I went to a club or a party and I had cocaine in my pocket, hey, I knew I would leave with a lady on my arm. . . . It was an instant success ticket with the ladies." Again, other members laughed and agreed, while another person added, "Yeah, you were cool when you had cocaine."

Doing cocaine with a group of people is one way to feel accepted; one woman who had dealt cocaine to support herself and her habit described how dealing made her feel important:

I was one of the few women dealers, and as I dealt at a higher and higher level there were all these people who hung around waiting to **score** coke for their customers, or just because they knew I was generous so they could always get turned on free. It was a power trip for me. Here I was being cool, having all this money and all these people around. It was a trip. I had instant friends and power (or so I thought at the time). It all seemed to revolve around me.

It seems ironic that most people who had originally been attracted to the drug because it seemed to offer group acceptance often end up either rejecting the group because they get so paranoid and edgy they can't deal with other people, or because they become so protective of their cocaine that they don't want to share it with anyone. But again, that's one of the symptoms and paradoxes of the disease.

After they've been clean for a while, people also realize that long after the fun of being with others was gone, they were still obsessively using cocaine, hoping to re-experience those good feelings but unable to get past the edgy paranoia that makes being around people uncomfortable and painful.

The group surrounding cocaine users sometimes disappears for another reason: The coke is gone. Some people can virtually smell cocaine, and when it's around, they're around; when the coke runs out, they're gone. These people, who will cozy up to a person who has cocaine, waiting for a cocaine handout, are referred to as "cocaine whores." These people can be men or women, and they can be from all walks of life. If you have cocaine around, they'll be there. Friends? Supporters? A support system? No, not really, because when the cocaine runs out, they're gone.

Another paradox of group involvement and cocaine usage is that, in order to get clean, many addicts have to separate from their "friends" who still use coke. As one man said,

I tried to go around Andy's house and he was friendly enough, but something was missing. Along about my third visit there he said, "You wouldn't mind if I did some coke, would you?" And I didn't think I would. But when I saw him chop up that coke and begin to lay out some lines like we always used to do, I just jumped up and got the hell out, I was afraid I couldn't have resisted if I saw those lines all laid out and ready to be snorted . . . later on I was thinking about it and realized that me and Andy, we used to get together all the time, but it was always about doing coke. I didn't have anything in common with him anymore. I guess you could say that when I stopped doing drugs, I grew out of him.

While some of my clients have been able to maintain old drug-related friendships, usually this happens only when the friends do not do drugs in front of them or do not come around when they're high. This usually happens with friends who were recreational or occasional users. On the other hand, if an addict's friends are all addicts, then the addict in recovery will have to find a new group of friends (preferably a group that is clean and sober). **Cocaine Anonymous**, **Alcoholics Anonymous**, **Narcotics Anonymous**, (Chemical Dependency) **Recovery Groups**, and **Alano Clubs** provide excellent places to meet other people who have common interests and who are willing to accept new members. These groups provide a healthier atmosphere than the drug-related groups, which had become a large part of the problem.

"IT WAS A GREAT WAY TO ESCAPE"

People also become involved with cocaine because it provides a great way to escape. Escape from what? From boredom, from life, from worries, from problems, mostly from "the same old shit." One woman said,

Cocaine allowed me to escape from my daily routine to an exciting feeling state. I could pretend I was a part of a more razzle-dazzle lifestyle. And that was exciting at first. I mean, I had never had a way to relate to that Hollywood glitter world (but I had always wanted to), and when I did cocaine I felt like I was. . . . I know that sounds crazy, but I enjoyed those fantasies. They were important to me, they made me feel important, something I could not do on a regular, day-to-day basis.

Cocaine does seemingly offer a respite from depression, shyness, boredom, the same old routine; it can be fun, at first, until it becomes a problem. Some people have found that cocaine could be a great escape when they didn't want to be a part of anything, when they wanted to drop out from their daily pressures.

Hey, when I was down I knew how to get up, I just had to get my pipe all ready and **fire it up**, it got so that I couldn't stand being down, not even mildly depressed, I had to escape that feeling, I had to get high . . . so I did.

People who use cocaine heavily often begin to use it alone, turning it into an isolating experience (escaping even more from any sort of interaction with people) instead of the social event it had been. Addicts have such a pervasive denial system that they do not recognize the transition for what it is: a movement from recreational to abusive or addictive cocaine use. Thus they continue to use, except that now they use and abuse the drug when they are alone. At that point, the cocaine reinforces the need to be alone, to be isolated, and not to be bothered; the cocaine serves as a "Do Not Disturb" sign. This isolation allows their own distorted reality to rule, effectively eliminating outside influences. As a result, they are more likely to block out any realistic views of what's happening, and indulge in their own self-serving or self-undermining views of reality.

"IT WAS A WAY TO SABOTAGE MY SUCCESS AND FLIRT WITH THE EDGE"

Sometimes people in treatment realize that cocaine abuse has been a way to play out their self-destructive tendencies, though they hadn't realized this while they were using. After they've been clean a few weeks, this issue tends to come up in therapy. In this dialogue "Ron" talks about how he sabotaged his success with drugs.

Ron: You know, I worked real hard to get where I was, real hard, and when I finally got there, to a more comfortable place financially, I started blowing it all on coke.

Therapist: Do you see any connections there between achieving what you wanted and starting to blow it with coke?

Ron: Financial; I was able to afford it.

Therapist: Anything else?

Ron: Like what?

Therapist: Did you deserve what you had?

Ron: That's a peculiar question, did I deserve it—I certainly worked real hard to get it.

Therapist: So you deserved it?

Ron: Well . . . yes and no . . .

Therapist: What's the "no" part?

Ron: What pops into my head is that my father always threatened me that I wouldn't "make it"; I kept coming up with money-making schemes in high school, but I had no follow-through, and he used to say that I took big gambles and always lost. Then he went and died while I was away at college.

Therapist: So, is some of you playing out that old routine that you'll ultimately blow it all and not amount to anything?

Ron: You know, I always wondered if he knew something about me that I didn't see. . . . He seemed so sure of himself . . . and so sure that I would always be on the brink but never quite make it.

Therapist: You know, in a crazy way then, you would be pleasing him by failing.

Ron: What?

Therapist: You'd be proving him right.

Ron: [Shuddering] Oh God, I hope I'm not doing that; then I'd be stuck failing.

Therapist: Well, even if you're not doing that consciously, it sounds like you might, on some level, believe him. And you're operating and building on that self-fulfilling prophecy of failure.

Ron: Oh shit, this is beginning to sound plausible in a crazy way.

Therapist: So what else could you do?

Ron: Succeed?

Therapist How?

Ron: Stay away from cocaine, for one. And give myself permission to prove to my father, once and for all, that I won't always sabotage myself with my own inaction or without thinking things through and having good follow through plans.

Therapist   Do you think you can do that?

Ron: I think so.

Therapist: Do you deserve it?

Ron: Damned right, that old man up there needs to know that I'm not such a wash-out.

This is an example of a client who let his father's ghost rule his life; he had an excuse to sabotage his own success. People can sabotage themselves by having an overwhelming desire to have it all now, instant success and instant recognition; or a feeling that, no matter what the consequences may be, "I worked so hard for the past ten years, I deserve a special treat right now!"

This is not to say that people have control over their addiction and become addicted because they have self-destructive tendencies. They become addicted because they are addicts—they are unable to control their usage, they continue in the face of negative effects, and they use compulsively. However, we can look at their tendencies to overdo and overindulge as patterns that will get them in trouble in different aspects of their lives.

When I discussed these tendencies with another client, Diane, she said, "You know, I always feel like a winner; I'm not a loser, yet here's something that makes me feel like a loser and I keep doing it, I just don't understand."

Therapist: Do you have any clues as to why you might be doing this?

Diane: No, not really . . . only I never got much encouragement when I was a kid. I felt like I had to do it all on my own, but I also felt like I could do it.

Therapist: It sounds like something was missing.

Diane: What do you mean?

Therapist   You say you knew you could make it, and you also knew you had to do it on your own.

Diane: Yeah, so what are you driving at?

Therapist: It seems like a lot for a little kid to know in her guts. . . . Sometimes the absence of adult or parental encouragement and support makes you feel like you don't really deserve it all.

Diane: Oh yeah?

Therapist: Yeah, it's like if your folks aren't backing you up, who's gonna?

Diane: Hmm . . .

Therapist: And somewhere along the line you had to discover it's a pretty powerful place out there—the real world.

Diane: You're right there.

Therapist: See how this sounds: You knew on some level that you would need support to get by in that powerful world. And when that support isn't there from the people it is supposed to be there from, you can unconsciously get the idea that you don't deserve it and you won't ever have it. So that although you feel consciously that you're a winner, unconsciously you feel "Oh no, I'm not going to make it, I don't have the support I need."

              And then you discovered a good escape from this internal battle, you discovered cocaine . . . and it made you feel good at first, real good, a real boost to that part of you that wants to have it now. But now your job's on the line . . . your other part—the part that knows deep down you don't have what it takes—is sinking from the weight of this addiction. You've just go to jump ship with this addiction, get on solid dry land, and reassess this internal conflict.

Diane: Whoa, I gotta think about that one for a while.

Therapist: Fine, think about it. I'm in no rush. . . .

People sabotage their success for all kinds of reasons: fear of success, fear of failure, old unresolved conflicts working on conscious or unconscious levels; intentional or unintentional actions that will assure failure are common. With some people cocaine and its effects feed directly into these tendencies. Therapy can help them sort out the whys and wherefores and come up with new options and choices. This is possible when people have stopped using the drug and can use their chemical-free brains to think clearly. But until then, the paradoxical effects of cocaine wreak havoc on a person's ability to cope with life and make effective decisions.

THE PARADOXICAL EFFECTS OF COCAINE

During a session of one of my recovery groups, members started listing all the reasons why they used cocaine. They discovered that all the original reasons were stated positively—It made me feel more social, It gave me the power to face things. Yet all these reasons were reversed over time as the drug and addiction took control. Then they became less social and primarily wanted to do their cocaine alone; they did not want to share the drug or the drug experience with anyone. The group members were very surprised at this discovery. One woman summed it up by saying, "I guess I was too high to notice."

Cocaine is a "quick-picker-upper" during initial phases of use, bringing you up when you feel down. The problem with using it to feel better is that when a person **crashes**—comes down from a cocaine high—life usually looks worse than it did before. The emotional let down is combined with a concept (borrowed from economics) called "relative deprivation," which makes the non-drug-induced reality that follows a drug-induced high seem worse. When you reexperience reality and compare it to the high feeling and state you had been in, reality seems worse—it is actually a new, lower state.

As a result, many people don't want to deal with being down, they'd rather be high. So they go for more coke, entering into a bouncing ball syndrome of crashing to the non-drug-induced state, which seems too low, and then trying to get high again to avoid what they are distortingly calling reality. With each successive bounce, the down state appears more grim and the illusion of that cocaine high seems much better; although in fact, at some point the addict stops getting relief from getting high; the cocaine-induced paranoia replaces the high, fun feelings. After a while, all states blend into one negative abyss.

Figure 1 illustrates this point. The area above the reality line represents good feelings—excitement, fun, euphoria; and the area below the reality line represents negative feelings—depression, edginess, irritability, paranoia, anger, and rage. Over time, cocaine use induces an artificially low emotional state, and eventually the cocaine will not even get a user to that euphoric up state, but will simply induce irritability, paranoia, and finally rage. The end result is an addict who seems to be in a permanent state of

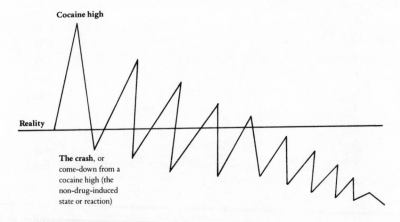

Figure 1 Cocaine-induced emotional states

doom and gloom. When addicts stop doing the drug, they snap back to reality within a few days, usually somewhat disoriented from having had a distorted view of reality for a period of time. But this disorientation also passes as they become readjusted to real life.

4. "I'm Not an Addict, I Just Use the Stuff a Lot"

It is very hard for people to judge their own degree of drug usage. Most people, especially abusers and addicts, underestimate their drug intake by about 50 percent; but even people who use recreationally often underestimate their usage. Reasons for underestimation vary. Recreational users know they don't have a problem, so they don't bother to pay attention. They know how they feel when they are doing cocaine and when they want to stop; and they do stop when they want to stop. They can easily refuse offers of cocaine and other drugs. Recreational users usually can estimate quite accurately how often they snort cocaine, and how much they have bought in the last year. In fact, recreational users can probably tell you about most of the cocaine purchases they have made in the last year.

One man who heard about my work with cocaine addiction asked me how much cocaine I thought was a safe amount to use. I replied, "None." He blanched and looked quite upset and asked, "Why do you say none?"

Therapist: Because it is so highly addictive I don't think it's worth the risk. They say only two in ten people who use cocaine will become addicted, but after hearing so many of those supposed two-in-ten stories, I don't think it's worth not knowing before hand if you are one of the unlucky twos.

Gene: Oh, I see . . . I was wondering, because I use cocaine sometimes.

Therapist: How often is sometimes?

Gene: Oh, maybe three times a year, with my wife, on special occasions.

Therapist: Is it really just three times a year?

Gene: Yes.

Therapist: Well, if that's all . . . and you've been doing that for how long?

Gene: Two years or so.

Therapist: That definitely falls into the recreational category. Just watch it, remember it is illegal, and make sure those "special occasions" don't start happening more often. Some people think getting through one hour is a special occasion and worth celebrating with a couple lines of coke.

Gene: [Laughing] Oh no, really, it's maybe three times a year.

RECREATIONAL USERS

Gene is definitely a recreational user. Even if we apply the usual underestimation formula of 50 percent less than actual usage and multiply his usage by two, six times a year would still be considered recreational.

A recreational user does cocaine only on an occasional basis. "Occasional," of course, is a relative term. To this man, it is three times a year. To someone else, it is at rock concerts; to others, it's before a party or only on Friday nights.

The timing for cocaine use is not the only factor that must be considered; the amount is important too. One client I saw for a brief period only did cocaine Friday nights, but each week he did two or three grams, making two or three frantic trips to his dealer a night. He was on automatic, unable to let a Friday night go by without doing cocaine. Each Friday night he used up at least half his paycheck and was unable to make ends meet. Even though he didn't want to use cocaine anymore because of the guilt, the terrible mood swings, and the waste of money, he was unable to stop. He only used once a week, but he was not a recreational user; he was what is called a binge addict.

A recreational user also has the ability to turn cocaine down easily when it is offered. Some people (for instance, people in the entertainment world) come into contact with cocaine on a daily basis; for these people to remain recreational users, they must turn cocaine down most of the time it's offered.

Recreational users will usually only use cocaine for a special occasion. It is savored as a fine champagne would be savored, and only bought for a celebration. It is not devoured as quickly as possible. Recreational users will snort cocaine calmly. They may be excited about getting it, but they won't purchase it frenetically, or nervously prepare and ingest all of it as quickly as possible. One recreational user told me:

I get half a gram every month or two. It lasts me the whole month or so. Every so often, I remember I have it and I go in and have a line or two, or I offer some to friends. Sometimes, I think about it and don't feel like it, so I don't use it. I just like the feeling I get from snorting a small line or two. More than that, my teeth get clenched and I feel too hyper so I stick with a real small amount. You know, I think my friends do more of it than me. They all laugh when they see how little I do, but I'm okay with that. I don't really understand why they do so much. It would make me too hyper. Maybe it doesn't affect them the way it does me. In any event, I can take it or leave it.

This woman is a recreational user. She uses on an irregular basis; she uses very little at a time, and turns down extra with no problem. She can take it or leave it. I would caution her, however, that if she continues to associate with people who are heavily into cocaine and she has it around all the time, she may very well begin to use more and move from being a recreational user to an abuser of cocaine. She is in a somewhat vulnerable position because of its constant availability. At this time, she uses irregularly, but not on special occasions, so she could be at risk if her irregular use becomes more regular and she begins to increase the amount she uses as her tolerance increases.

True recreational users will only use cocaine on an occasional basis. They will be able to turn it down easily and will be able to use some of the cocaine available and leave some for another time. They will not feel a compulsive need to use it all up at once, in one sitting. It is not difficult to tell if someone is a recreational user, but the distinction between an abuser and an addict is often much harder to make; it is actually based on a matter of degrees of severity.

People who come into contact with cocaine frequently may find it easy to kid themselves into thinking. "Oh, I'm okay; look at her. She uses all the time. I'm only doing it a few times a week." A few times a week, however, is no longer recreational. It is being used too regularly to be considered recreational. People in this category find it harder and harder to turn down, and have to rationalize their usage by saying, "But I turned it down earlier today." When turning cocaine down becomes a real struggle and it's easier to say "yes" than "no." they've moved from being recreational users to becoming, at best, abusers.

ABUSERS

Abusive cocaine users use cocaine on a chronic and frequent basis. They still pay their bills, but may no longer have the money to go to the movies or out to eat at nice restaurants very often. As their abuse gets worse and they start sliding over into addiction, they will be more lax, tending to make minimum payments and falling behind with some bills.

Monetary amounts cannot be assigned to these categories, because they are relative to a person's income. A person who grosses $25,000 and buys a half a gram every week to ten days may not look like someone with a serious problem to a person using two to three grams a day. Yet, that person is spending $55 every ten days, or $1,980 a year. Considering that a single person only sees about $13,000 of every $25,000 earned, that is a good chunk— and it doesn't even count the amount that person will spend on alcohol and other drugs to cut the edge off the coke high. Such people are not going to be able to afford a lot of recreational activities such as movies, concerts, or eating out. Their social life or good times will revolve around cocaine and other cocaine users.

People who associate good times with cocaine are abusive users. Abusive users infrequently, if ever, turn down cocaine when it is offered. Cocaine abusers use cocaine regularly on a chronic and frequent basis, looking forward to their next usage even as they are snorting or freebasing their present **stash**. People who abuse cocaine associate it with "good times," because they don't have any extra money to have good times in other ways, nor do they really want to.

If you were to observe a cocaine abuser, you would see erratic mood swings from a rather frenetic good feeling to depression and low productivity. The work produced during that frenetic-good-feeling mood would soon begin to look very sloppy and unorganized. Abusers tend to think they are doing good work when they're high, because at times they feel so in control and their denial systems are so strong.

Abusers will begin to miss appointments because they "overslept." Why have they overslept? They may have been up snorting cocaine all night, or have a hangover from all the booze they drank in an effort to come down from the cocaine and fall asleep.

When people begin to abuse cocaine, their friends who are not heavily involved will notice that their friend seems to be "changing." Those changes may include mood swings, increased irritability, irresponsibility, increased sense of paranoia, inconsistent behavior (such as saying one thing and doing something entirely different), and sloppier personal habits. A careful observer will definitely see these types of emotional and behavorial changes.

ADDICTS

The lines of distinction between addictive cocaine use and abusive cocaine use are hazy, at best. With addiction, all the symptoms outlined above are intensified. Addicts begin to tell elaborate stories to cover their tracks. They need to develop explanations for why they are always broke or having financial problems. If they are snorting cocaine, they have to develop chronic sinus problem stories to explain their running noses. If they are shooting cocaine, they won't wear short sleeves. If they are freebasing, they will develop a cough and lung problems.

Addicts often develop a fairly elaborate "reality" that they believe. They have to do this to justify their continued drug usage in the face of negative effects. One client told me of an incident that was one of her lowest points, and which led her to begin a serious recovery program:

Kathy: I was out with this friend of mine, someone who I had always done cocaine with. We were having a few drinks and I said, "Want to come to my house? I have some good coke." The fact of the matter was . . . I can't believe I did this . . . and I can't believe I'm even telling you this.

Therapist: Go on, you're doing fine.

Kathy: It's so hard, even now to admit, but I've got to be honest if I'm going to stay clean and sober. I got this girl over to my house and I got frantic. I didn't really have any coke. I'd been broke. She had bought me the drinks and I wanted to give her something. I *wanted* to have cocaine. I went into my bedroom and remembered I had some cut, you know, what I used to use to cut cocaine before I'd sell it. I brought that out, chopped it up and laid out the lines. She took one hit and said, "What the hell is this?" I said, "It's coke!" She said, "What? Are you crazy or something? That's not cocaine." I just broke down. I was never so mortified. I had tried to pass off this cut as cocaine. I knew I was addicted then. I knew that was as low as I wanted to go.

Addicts will construct lies and believe them because they have to. This woman's pride was hurt. She wanted to repay her friend for the drinks. Before her drug usage had gotten out of control, she had had a lot of money and had been very generous with her drugs. She couldn't accept being broke and not having any drugs. In fact, she said to me, "I really couldn't see why people would like me if I didn't have money or drugs." Because she denied her current situation, she created even more pain by her elaborate lies that began to backfire when she couldn't even keep them straight anymore.

Addicts lose all touch with their previous priorities in life. Prior to becoming addicted, they may have held a job, had a family, and put those priorities above more self-indulgent things, like spending the family's food money on drugs. Recovering addicts often say,

If you had told me I would be basing coke I had bought with money that should have been for my babies' dinner, I'd have killed you. But I was, and I just couldn't see it. I was blinded by the drug. My marriage to the drug was much stronger and more important than my marriage to my wife.

Addicts put their drug of choice on a pedestal, higher than anything else in their lives. Addicts will do anything, including leaving their families hungry or not buying their children Christmas presents, just so they can get their drugs. An addict's partner has a very tough time knowing where reality ends and where the lies composing the addict's reality begin. When a partner starts feeling confused, hurt, and emotionally unstable from trying to keep up with the other partner's ups and downs, he or she needs help also. The partner needs to try to do an **intervention**, or get a professional to come in and organize an intervention to see if the addict will go for help; simultaneously, the partner must also begin to get his or her life back in order.

Cocaine addiction can become very dangerous, not just for the user, but also for those around the user. A cocaine addict is likely to develop cocaine psychosis, and can be very paranoid, even violent. The following story shows how far this can go.

My co-therapist and I treated a couple, "Rick" and "Nina," who were in crisis. Rick had badly beat Nina because he was sure she had stolen his money. In fact, he had been on a ten-day freebasing run and had gone through all of his money. He couldn't believe he had gone through $12,000, so he was sure she had taken it.

Nina was advised to go to a woman's shelter until Rick calmed down; but unfortunately, she wouldn't leave him to protect herself. She believed she had to take care of him; in her mind, that did not include protecting herself and him from his violent outbursts. (She had also been freebasing with him; not as much, they both said, but more than enough to distort her thinking.)

We were able to calm them down and they left, against our advice, before we felt they were able to stay out of trouble. Sure enough, they went out, got some more coke on credit, and based all of it. Rick went into another uncontrollable rage, ransacked their apartment, and then attacked Nina.

She returned to us with more bruises, and finally agreed to go to a friend's house for a few weeks. She kept saying, "But he doesn't usually do this. I don't understand. He loves me, why did he hurt me? He promised he would never hurt me." I tried to explain to her that cocaine addiction and cocaine psychosis are not controllable unless you stop taking the drugs. Until they both eliminated cocaine from their lives, they were guaranteed to have more trouble.

Addicts are people who use cocaine (or any other drug) in an uncontrollable way; their usage is compulsive and continuous, despite obvious adverse effects. Most addicts I see in treatment have lost all or most of their money. They have lost relationships, families, jobs, homes, or cars. They have very little left except a basic survival sense, and even that is often questionable. Many addicts wait to come to treatment until they are so low there is only one direction left: up.

Yet, I've seen some who have to keep rediscovering new lows because they can't stay convinced that they must give up all drugs. Their denial, their fear of change, their fear of sobriety, and their fears of feeling their own feelings are so huge that the only way they know to handle those fears is to use again.

It becomes a vicious cycle. I have to let people like that go. I give them my card, and let them know I'll be here and glad to help them when they are ready, but that I don't want to make it easier for them to think they are helping themselves when they are not ready to face reality, and I don't want to watch them die. Some call again, when they are more ready, and then we can work.

Cocaine addicts seem pretty crazy to straight people. They have frequent and erratic mood swings, from way up to way down. They appear irresponsible, forgetful, and very self-centered; they go from self-deprecation to an outrageous "greater-than-thou" attitude. Cocaine addicts also tend to be snobbish about "those alcoholics and dope fiends," and see themselves as different from those people. Cocaine addicts may also exhibit all three stages of cocaine psychosis at various times, ranging from irritability, to mild paranoia, to more serious paranoia and uncontrollable rages. They will lie, cheat, embezzle, and steal for their drugs; people who have never done those kinds of things before will do them for cocaine.

All these symptoms are reversible for addicts who make the decision to enter recovery programs, and to live drug-free lives. This recovery process can be an exciting challenge for both addict and therapist, but it is always underscored by the knowledge that the addict who continues to use is heading for death: from an overdose; from the presence of bad cuts, such as too much lidocaine; or cancer of the lungs.

Addicts who continue to use are gambling in a high-stakes, no-win game. It's up to them to walk away from the table and take another kind of chance, one that is immensely frightening to most addicts: that life can be sweeter without drugs. "But what if it isn't?" addicts often ask me anxiously. I reply, "What have you got to lose in trying?"

5. Does He or Doesn't He? Only His Dealer Knows for Sure

It is not hard to detect cocaine abuse if you know what to watch for. Sooner or later, frequent users of cocaine will begin to show telltale changes in their emotional behavior and work habits, which may also be accompanied by physiological symptoms.

GENERAL SIGNS TO WATCH FOR

When a person first starts using cocaine there are a few signs one can watch for, but they are not as marked as those that will appear later, if the person abuses or is addicted to cocaine. A person who uses cocaine will have enlarged pupils while the cocaine is actively working. This may last from about five to forty minutes, depending upon the potency of the dose. After snorting the drug the person may have a runny nose with a watery discharge. Some people react strongly to the withdrawal of cocaine and become depressed and irritable as soon as the drug wears off, (not everyone has this emotional response, especially not every recreational user).

The more frequent and regular the usage, the more signs one can watch for. Unfortunately, there are no glaring signs that say, "Help me, I'm in trouble and not realizing it yet, so help now before it gets too bad!" A person who uses cocaine heavily will begin to exhibit behavioral, physiological, and emotional changes. The user becomes adept at covering up these changes, denying their existence, and explaining them away. It is up to concerned family, friends, and partners (co-dependents or cos) to avoid getting sucked into the addict's reality. **Al-Anon**, **Nar-Anon** and a therapist specializing in chemical dependency can be very helpful to significant others. If you suspect that a person may be using too much cocaine, it is important to get educated about the drug and about addiction in general so you can deal with the problem effectively; sometimes your only choice is to deal with your own feelings and reactions to it.

EMOTIONAL SYMPTOMS

MOOD SWINGS

People who use cocaine regularly will experience and exhibit frequent mood swings. One minute they will be up—excited, energetic, happy; and before you know what happened, they are depressed, low, don't want to do anything, and are very unhappy and irritable. Frequently cos ask themselves "What happened?" or "What did I do?" The co can do nothing and has done nothing. Cocaine and the disease of addiction have done it all.

Addicts grow to love the cocaine high, that initial rush they first felt when using cocaine. They continue to search it out, time after time, long after cocaine has ceased to get them high. Each time they purchase cocaine they anxiously anticipate the remembered rush. Instead, they experience the crash, the irritability, and later the paranoia and maybe even uncontrollable rages. Time after time, they will deny the reality and stubbornly do more; they are looking for that illusory high, but feel worse and worse, and act miserable enough that others get caught up in it.

This cycle of misery and desperation is a little-acknowledged reality shared by many cocaine addicts. In a group of cocaine addicts who are just beginning to consider a recovery program, stories that glorify cocaine abound. Each person has a more outrageous story than the previous teller. "Remember when . . . ?" or "There was this incredible time . . . " or "The first time I got off on cocaine, man, it was just too fine. . . . " People tend to minimize and keep to themselves stories about the time "My heart was racing so fast I was sure it was going to jump out of my chest and I was going to die."

Minimizing negative realities of cocaine abuse is part of the denial process. It allows users to go on using and abusing and having "fun." They can justify their fun with tales of cocaine glory. During treatment I do not allow people to revel in their cocaine stories; instead, we look at the suppressed negative aspects and the scary realities of cocaine addiction.

DISTORTIONS OF REALITY

I am often amazed at how strongly people can hold on to their distorted views of reality, unable to let go of their illusions. One young man I worked with had trouble giving up his self-made glory of being one of the first basers in San Francisco. He kept talking about all the people he taught how to base:

I am the acknowledged king of basing where I live. They know when they want good **blow** where to go. I've always had it, always. That's how people know me. They've seen me like that for twelve years. And now I'm trying to stop. It's hard. They're still coming round, looking . . . so I'm doing real well, I'm only doing half a gram a day. That's good man. I'm used to basing two, three grams a day, easy.

This man only came to a few sessions and then would not respond to phone calls or messages left at work. It was not surprising, because he was so attached to his role. He was too proud of that to consider stepping down from his self-appointed "king of basers" status, which allowed him to deny his problem and continue to enjoy his elevated position within his drug-oriented circle of friends. And what did enjoyment look like to him? He talked of feeling paranoid a lot, of being so edgy at work that he was having trouble relating to other people. Enjoyment was, in fact, watching his life become more and more unmanageable.

DENIAL

One of the most frightening emotional changes for an outsider or a co is the tremendous build up of defenses called denial.

Addicts construct elaborate tales to justify their habit and its consequences. Denial is frightening to a co, because often he or she will feel an undercurrent of uneasiness, but cannot pinpoint what is happening or why. The co may know the user is in trouble, but is apt to believe excuses—after all, stress too can cause erratic behavior. For many who are unfamiliar with drug abuse, this may be the last possibility considered. Thus the co lives in a fearful and powerless position, knowing something is wrong, but not knowing what it is or how to deal with it. Until the problem is acknowledged and dealt with, the co suffers, indirectly, from the same problems.

One woman told me the following story about her boyfriend:

He was acting crazy and pretending everything was fine. I tried to agree, to live like he did, but he was so moody and so unpredictable. Life with him got harder and harder, more and more painful; till I got this aching feeling in my gut, like I had been kicked one too many times. But he had never hurt me, physically; so at first I thought something was wrong with me, that I couldn't take stress. But then one day I knew I had to get out of the relationship for my own self-preservation. By then I knew he was doing too much cocaine, and he had promised me he would cut down. I believed him. But life was still too hard. I tried to get him to go for help. I told him I'd stay with him if he went. He said he would, but kept putting it off. Something else always came up first.

Finally, one weekend he went on a binge and I called some of his friends to come over and help me do an intervention. I just knew I needed help. He was acting so paranoid, he accused me of betraying him, of being a bitch, of not understanding anything, of letting him down. Mostly he told me I was betraying him and then he stormed out before his friends got there.

That was it for me. Something snapped. I loved him, but I had to survive. I called Al-Anon and talked to a woman there. That helped a lot. It gave me the strength to say, "I don't want to be involved in this craziness anymore." Maybe if he had gone for some treatment . . . but I saw the pattern. He would give it lip service when he thought I would leave. He really wasn't going to do it, not for himself and not for me. So that was pretty much the end.

He tried to come back a few weeks later, but I wouldn't let him. My guts were just beginning to stop aching. And I had to survive.

It was hard, because, like I said, I loved the man. I learned later that I loved the man, not the addict, but he didn't have faith enough in himself to be the man and let go of the addict. I still feel sad about that. It's such a waste of a human being. It really is.

I was angry at him for a long time, angry because he wouldn't get better; but that's his choice. In a crazy way I thought I could help him or force him to make that choice, but now I know that was crazy thinking on my part. So I've stopped, and even the anger has largely subsided. I think that's a sign that I'm getting healthier. And that feels good. I tell you though, it hasn't been easy unhooking myself.

One lawyer explained to me how he denied his cocaine problem:

I knew it was bad when I was straight. I knew it was breaking up my marriage. The financial limitations that it caused . . . I was running out of excuses I could tell my wife for why I was always broke. I can't tell you how many times she said, "You're acting different," or she asked, "What's wrong?" I kept telling her it was stress from work and not to worry. But I tell you, as soon as I walked into the bathroom and snorted a few lines I forgot my remorse, my financial responsibilities, her worried face; I had it under control. It [cocaine] gave me the confidence to walk into a courtroom and face a judge and jury and argue my case effectively. It really did, at first.

And long after it ceased to have that effect and I was getting scared "they'd" find out, I still kept doing cocaine. In fact, I started doing more, getting it from different **connections**, trying desperately to feel in control, when in fact my life was crumbling around me. But I didn't see it for so long. It's scary how long it took me to see it.

So I now know how capable I am of deceiving myself and other people, it's crazy and I don't like it. But I don't think I would have done it without the cocaine.

This lawyer was able to hide his cocaine habit from his unsuspecting wife for over three years. In fact, even as he was beginning to enter his recovery program he was not yet able to tell her about his addiction. I hope some day he will, because part of a recovery program entails making amends, telling people about the addiction, and apologizing for what he or she did as a result of the active drug addiction.

ADDICTION AS A FAMILY DISEASE

The addict's craziness affects other people. It's catching. In fact, addiction is called a family disease—because family members often work at least as hard as the addict to make a crazy situation seem sane and normal. That is part of the addict's defensive behavior; the addict tries to defend against all accusations. The ability to make up explanations, stories, and excuses, and to reverse the blame, is incredible. One woman told me,

He used to blame me for misplacing money. And I believed him. I was sure I had either misplaced it or mismanaged it. But goddamn it; he was stealing it. Our household money that was supposed to pay for our food and weekly expenses was going up his nose. Did I feel like a jerk when I found out!

Here is a perfect example. This woman's first reaction to the discovery that her husband had been stealing their money was to feel like a jerk, to blame herself for being naive and getting "taken." She had internalized and come to believe her husband's accusations, which made him innocent and put the blame on her. It took her a while to get angry at him. It was easier, at first, to blame herself, which is also crazy addiction-affected thinking.

Ultimately, addicts may also alienate their non-drug-abusing friends, because these friends will not tolerate more and more far-fetched alibis. Eventually, they will tire of the mood swings, the irritability, the jumpiness, the growing paranoia and ability to blame others. The more addicts blame others and begin to believe these accusations, the more they will withdraw from their support system.

Addicts may replace old **straight** friends with a new group of friends who also do a lot of drugs, (although, eventually, cocaine usage usually turns from being a social experience to a more isolated experience). After more time has passed, this self-imposed isolation becomes somewhat necessary financially, as addicts produce less and need more cocaine; but it also may be an attempt to minimize the paranoid thinking that gets triggered by being with other people. These paranoid thoughts may run along the lines of, "That's my coke, goddamn it," or "They sure are generous with my coke," or "Look at those giant lines they're putting out," or "They're using too much of my coke." These thoughts lead addicts to withdraw even from these drug-using friends, preferring to be alone with their cocaine.

COCAINE PSYCHOSIS

The most extreme emotional changes fall under the heading of cocaine psychosis. This temporary condition can look just like a classic psychotic break, complete with paranoid delusions, auditory and visual hallucinations, uncontrollable rages, and loss of reality.

Cocaine psychosis has three stages. The first, irritability and depression, is experienced by most users in their crash from the drug. Stage two is characterized by more erratic and marked mood swings and paranoia, and is more apt to be experienced by abusers and addicts. Stage three is similar to stage two, except symptoms are exaggerated and may present additional behaviors: auditory or visual hallucinations and uncontrollable rages. Addicts themselves often wonder about their own behavior, but usually deny its existence when they are high or still trying to justify their habits. Cocaine psychosis usually quickly subsides if the person stops using cocaine. Antipsychotic drugs may need to be prescribed in small doses for a few days for someone who is experiencing an acute stage-three reaction.

Cocaine use, abuse, and addiction is such a new phenomenon that new findings roll in all the time. For years it was thought that cocaine was only psychologically addictive, but new evidence suggests that cocaine is also physiologically addictive. Some people who have used excessive amounts of cocaine do seem to experience sleep disturbances for a few days to a few weeks after getting off the drug. They can be very nervous and have trouble controlling their anxiety. We do not yet know if these withdrawal symptoms are emotionally or physically based, although evidence is beginning to suggest they may be physically based. We do know that these emotional changes affect a person's personal life and job performance.

Former users also experience what has been called "drug hunger," an involuntary craving for the drug often accompanied by strong images of purchasing and using the drug. These drug cravings can persist for months. People relate drug dreams from which they wake up frightened, because they used cocaine in their dreams or refused it in their dreams. These types of reactions are upsetting to people in the beginning stages of recovery. I always reassure them that they are natural reactions and they can expect them to persist for some time, although they may fade in intensity.

Some people experience "drug hunger" for days, weeks, months, and sometimes, intermittently, for years. Dreams also tend to recur for years, and people simply learn to accept them. Some of the clients I work with say they have trouble sleeping at first and feel anxious. I try to tell them that's a natural response to removing the drug from their system and it too will pass. Sometimes I make a systematic muscle relaxation tape for them to listen to whenever they need to relax. Their anxiety seems to pass as they get excited about their recovery and all the new options they begin to see as real possibilities.

WORK BEHAVIOR

ATTENDANCE

Sometimes an employer will notice that a particular employee arrives late for work on a fairly consistent basis. Absences from work begin to increase. On some days the employee may not even call into work with an explanation. In these cases the person has probably stayed up all night snorting cocaine and overslept in the morning. If the employee snorted, freebased, or injected too much cocaine and began to feel irritable and jumpy, he or she may also have drunk alcohol excessively to relieve these symptoms or taken a few Valiums and then slept in with a hangover. In the

morning, feeling remorseful or even wanting to deny what occurred, the user won't bother to call in to work. Another possibility is the person may have a bad hangover and be afraid his or
her voice will "give it away." In this case the lesser of two evils
is just not to call in at all and simply show up the next day.

A person in this stage of denial constructs elaborate cover
stories, going to great lengths to try to make strange behavior
seem to be a normal response to a peculiar situation. One client
said:

> I told my supervisor that my mother was sick so many times that I was
> scared she would get sick and it would be my fault. I had nightmares
> about it; but that didn't stop me from telling stories about her bad heart.
> The stories got more and more grandiose, but I only realized that after
> I stopped using. At the time I thought I was entitled to have a sick
> mother, it made my life easier.

JOB PERFORMANCE

Abusers or addicts have poor self-judgment as the quality and
quantity of their work output begins to vary. This poor judgment
is a symptom of how desperately they try to cover up their tracks.
They produce while they can, while they feel creative—that is,
when they have cocaine in their system—and need **down time**
to re-energize when the coke wears off. Abusers may appear
listless at work and not be able to produce at the pace they used
to. Sometimes they will get a spurt of energy and produce a lot
of work. Users tend to think such work is brilliant, though closer
inspection by another employee usually shows that the quality is
not as good as the abuser is capable of producing. Abusers may
recognize this when they are not high, and may then wonder
what happened to their brilliant ideas. In a still more futile
attempt to produce at work, addicts may begin to make frequent
trips to the bathroom to snort coke or even to fix more cocaine.

Abusers and addicts become much more irritable and agitated
on the job. They do not take criticism well and will probably
appear very defensive and even hostile at times—and then they

withdraw. An employer could easily mistake a lot of these behaviors for classic burn-out signs. Indeed, they are similar, and there is an overlap in characteristics; yet in this case they are burn-out signs from doing too much cocaine, and not from doing too much work.

If these signs persist after the employee takes a few days off, a trip to the Employee Assistance Department (where an employee can speak with a counselor confidentially and be referred for help), or a call to a drug specialist from a local inpatient or outpatient drug program might be helpful. Many lives and a lot of productivity could be saved if people erred on the side of questioning whether their employee's mood swings and periodic frenetic behavioral output might be drug or alcohol-related, rather than assuming they're "just caused by something at home" or by job burn-out.

PHYSIOLOGICAL SYMPTOMS

Some of these burn-out signs have physiological as well as emotional and behavioral symptoms. Frequent users of cocaine begin to exhibit an array of physiological symptoms. Chronic sinus problems (frequent sniffling and a drippy nose) may suddenly appear. If a person claims allergies all year long (and previously only had them in the spring or summer), check for other emotional or productivity changes. Frequent colds, where the only symptom is a runny nose, could also be a telltale sign. People who snort too much coke can actually perforate their nasal membrane, resulting in both nostrils being connected.

Cocaine use leads to appetite loss. A person who uses cocaine regularly in an abusive or addictive fashion often suffers a weight loss, though this weight loss may not be present if an individual uses alcohol to cut the **edge** of coming off cocaine. If a person is using other drugs (such as Valium or heroin) to cut the edge, a marked appetite and weight loss may be present. People who use cocaine a lot often become malnourished because they aren't eating enough—they eat on the run, when they feel like it, and what they eat may not be nutritional. Malnourishment also affects a person's moods and behavior, exaggerating the negative and erratic consequences of cocaine abuse. Often an abuser will also eat a lot of sugar products because they give an extra added boost. These poor eating habits exacerbate all the other negative effects described in this chapter.

A person who injects cocaine will probably always wear long-sleeved shirts to cover the needle marks or **tracks**. These look like tiny red dots unless they become abscessed, producing large lumps under the skin. In beginning infectious stages, these lumps can have open, pussy sores.

A person who freebases cocaine excessively may develop lung problems that appear to have asthmatic-type symptoms. Researchers call this condition "cocaine lung," but the phenomenon is so new that long-term effects are still a mystery. Basers often develop persistent bad coughs. More serious problems can and do develop, and these will be discussed in the next chapter.

6. Watch Out: Dangers of Cocaine

Cocaine is a very dangerous drug. It is dangerous to one's emotional and physical well-being, and it can kill. During the 1960s speed—amphetamines—became very popular, and drug specialists became alarmed as the popularity quickly spread across America. An educational campaign that featured alarming but realistic facts about speed was launched. Posters proclaiming "Speed Kills" appeared across the nation. The educational campaign was effective, and the popularity of speed declined. Now we need to learn from that campaign and begin to educate people that cocaine also kills. Yes, cocaine kills; and you do not have to use enormous quantities to die from this drug.

Elsewhere in this book we have examined the various emotional reactions a person experiences. In this chapter we will examine the more serious reactions, which usually call for medical or psychiatric intervention. We will look at the physical and emotional components of cocaine psychosis, and we will look at all the physical reactions that cocaine can cause. Many of these negative effects are ignored or simply not attributed to cocaine. Maybe if more people knew about the negative consequences of using cocaine, fewer people would start to use it, and its mystique could be measured against its painful reality.

Let's begin by examining the behavior of monkeys and their experiences with cocaine. In one experiment, researchers set up conditions so that the monkeys were taught that by pressing one bar they would receive food and by pressing another they would receive cocaine. They could have unlimited supplies of either food or cocaine; all they had to do was press the appropriate bar. What happened? They continued to press the bar that yielded cocaine, ignoring the bar that yielded food, until they died from convulsions. Clearly, the cocaine became more important to them than food. Even in the face of starvation and the breakdown of their bodily functions, the monkeys preferred cocaine to food.

In a different experiment, monkeys were given a choice of receiving a high dose of cocaine along with an electric shock, or a low dose of cocaine without an electric shock. Monkeys don't like electric shocks; yet to get the cocaine, they accepted these shocks. After these results, researchers wanted to see how far monkeys would go to receive cocaine. In another experiment researchers kept making the monkeys press the bar more and more times in order to receive one dose of cocaine. The monkeys stayed and pressed the bar up to 12,800 times before they received one dose of cocaine. This shows perseverance in monkeys, and it also clearly demonstrates addictive behavior.

At the University of California Medical School in San Francisco, cocaine-related experiments were performed with rats. Rats were taught to go through mazes that had three openings; one contained food, one contained other rats, and one contained cocaine. The experiment was set up to examine the motivational qualities of some basic drives—hunger and sex as opposed to the drive for cocaine. As with the monkeys, cocaine seemed to be the ultimate reinforcer for the rats. They would run the mazes, find the food, and turn away; running another way in the maze they would find the rats, and snub them also. They wanted the cocaine. Even when the researchers changed the position of the reinforcers, the rats still went for the cocaine, rejecting the food and possibility of sex. The rats' behavior, like that of the monkeys, shows that they had become addicted to cocaine. Though human beings share that addictive potential with rats and monkeys, we are capable of reasoned thought. Given the necessary information, people can make some choices before they begin to use cocaine.

I don't know any cocaine addict who began by saying, "Oh wow, I'm going to become a cocaine addict." No, they all started pretty much the same, with a curiosity and probably some anticipatory excitement. They all believed they were using a harmless drug and they were going to have fun.

So how do so many people get hooked? Addiction is a disease that occurs when a person continues to use a substance in an uncontrolled and compulsive way, despite negative effects. Most important, addiction is not the result of a weak will or a lack of discipline or a poor character or a sagging backbone. It is a disease. When a person get diabetes nobody says, "You blew it. Why weren't you stronger?" When a person gets cancer you don't say, "What the hell did you do that for? If you had been stronger you wouldn't have it." And in turn, when it comes time for those people to get treatment, you don't say "Oh, try to be strong; try it without insulin." Or, "You don't really need chemotherapy; just stay away from cancer-causing foods like saccharin and you'll be fine." No, you tell these people to get treatment. If they have serious cases or are terminal or their disease is going to affect their personal and work lives, friends, family, or fellow workers may seek some help in adjusting to the changes in their lives caused by living or working with a person who is going through massive changes.

That is all part of treatment for a physical disease, and it is also true for addiction. It is a very real disease and it can be treated. Left untreated, addiction, like cancer and diabetes, is a chronic and ultimately terminal disease.

With treatment, an addict can live a full and very rich life, but without it he or she is almost assured of dying an early death. And that is perhaps one of the craziest components of the addictive disease: It is the only disease whose victims fight like hell against getting well. In treating addiction, you are initially fighting not only the disease itself, but also the addict's self-destructiveness (resulting from disease-produced denial), which encourages the addict to seek the very substances that will trigger the disease. Addiction therefore needs a continuous treatment or recovery program to prevent relapses from occuring.

Addiction is also frightening to those around the addict because it is a misunderstood disease, long veiled by the stereotype of the addict as a low-life or a skid-row type. We don't want to think of our successful accountant as an addict. We certainly don't want to think that the doctor who treats all our ailments might be an addict! The stereotype says that nice people aren't addicts; but that's just not true. Lots of nice people are addicts. They didn't ask for the disease; they just got it. And now they have to live with it. It is sad that addicts should have to fight the general public's outdated and untrue stereotypes in addition to fighting their own disease.

When I talk to addicts about their recovery, I tell them that recovery is a life-and-death issue. If they do not stop using and begin to take some concrete steps to make sure that they won't start using again, they are probably going to die from medical complications arising from their active addiction, or they will eventually overdose. I point out to them that there are not many old active addicts, they usually die rather young. One of my clients said to me (after being clean for about eight months and in a full recovery program):

For me, starting to use again is not a life-and-death issue, because I'm not afraid of dying. For me, my recovery is very important and using is much more scary when I look at the good life I have now and remember the horribly painful life I used to have. That's the issue for me. And that's what I'm afraid of; I'm afraid that if I start using again I won't die, and I'll just live the horrible existence I lived before. That's why my recovery is so important to me.

Addiction is a disease that requires an entire change in one's lifestyle to arrest its more dangerous effects. What I have seen suggests that people who do make the necessary changes—giving up all drugs, being in a recovery program, exercising, eating well, and in general learning how to live a healthy life—experience a marked difference in the quality of their life and are a lot happier than they were when they were actively using. As one woman I was working with said, "I wish I could have found all this out without getting in trouble with drugs so I could still enjoy a glass of wine with a good dinner. But if that's all I have to sacrifice in order to feel as good and alive as I feel, I guess it's not so bad."

Like alcoholics, cocaine addicts have to remember and not get cocky and think they have their addiction "licked" and become remiss with their recovery programs, because they always run a risk of using again. If they keep up with their recovery programs, they will be able to avoid all the dangers discussed in the rest of this chapter. If they don't keep up with a recovery program, they'll have trouble staying clean and sober.

PHYSIOLOGICAL EFFECTS OF COCAINE

Unlike the mixed bag of emotional effects produced by cocaine, which range from euphoria to dysphoria, the physiological effects of cocaine are mostly negative, ranging from irritations of the nasal membrane to death by acute cocaine poisoning and cocaine overdose. People are generally pretty surprised to hear that you can die from a cocaine overdose, probably because cocaine has enjoyed such a mystical reputation that the realities and consequences of its use are just not known or acknowledged. To understand how cocaine can so severely damage a person's physiological system, we need to know more about how cocaine operates and what parts of the body cocaine affects.

Cocaine works directly on the brain. This takes about three minutes by snorting cocaine, about 14 seconds by shooting, and about six seconds by freebasing. Once the cocaine reaches the brain, it acts as a block to a lot of normal brain cell activity. It affects the activity of the nerve cells that send messages to all parts of the body: messages like when to eat, when to sleep, and when to breathe. When these messages get blocked, basic bodily functions begin to break down.

In addition to blocking these essential messages, cocaine also has vasoconstrictive qualities—it causes the veins to constrict (decreasing the diameter of the veins), thereby building up the blood pressure. These vasoconstrictive qualities have proved useful in certain eye and nose surgeries, but they can also be very dangerous. Because when the effects of cocaine wear off, the blood pressure goes from an artificially elevated high to an artificial low, and that sudden drop can prove very dangerous and sometimes fatal.

Let's look at all this in more detail. If a person's blood pressure has been elevated high enough (from the vasoconstrictive effects of cocaine) and then dropped low enough when those effects wear off, death can occur. The key word here is "enough"—how much is "enough"? We do not know, and that is one of the dangerous realities of cocaine that users ignore. When they consciously get high, they do not know that they are actually playing a dangerous game of Russian roulette.

Along with narrowing the blood vessels, which clearly affects both the heart and circulatory systems, other risks are heart palpitations, angina (severe pain around the heart), arrhythmia (irregular heartbeat), and heart attack. One client told me about a time when his heart was beating so fast and so loudly that he thought it would jump out of his body; he said he was scared to death. When he tried to get up from the chair so he could call to buy more cocaine (to thereby get rid of his fears), he found that he couldn't move; his right side was paralyzed. Then he got even more scared. The paralysis was short-lived, lasting only a few hours, though it took a couple of weeks for him to get his full range of motion back. Unfortunately, during those weeks he "forgot" his terror and went back to cocaine. When I asked him how he could do that after what he had experienced, he said, "I just didn't think about it; I consciously blocked it out, saying 'but I'm okay now,' and then went for more of what I knew to do when I was in need of something—I'd go get some more cocaine." This is a great example of crazy addictive thinking.

Over time, snorting cocaine can do great damage to the nose. Initially, cocaine will just irritate the nasal membrane. Later, with continued usage, the irritation will become more severe and the cells will be damaged, ulcerate, and eventually die. When the nasal membrane is beginning to be damaged, the person will appear to have a stuffy or runny nose. The mucous will be very watery. When the condition becomes more severe, the user will have difficulty breathing; eventually, breathing through the nose will become impossible. A person who continues to snort cocaine will eventually disintegrate the wall dividing the halves of the nose (the septum); and in very extreme cases, the perforation grows so large that the septum will collapse completely, leaving no wall between the nostrils. Plastic surgeons are being called on more and more frequently to rebuild this wall and create a new septum.

Freebasing cocaine has its own set of negative effects. It can cause minor lung irritations, and a sore chest, neck, and cheeks. It also produces swollen glands on the floor of the mouth and a wispy, raspy voice. Over time, the cocaine can cause permanent damage to the vocal cords. Doctors are beginning to report that prolonged and chronic use can cause serious deterioration of the lung tissue, which is being called "smokers lung." Though freebasing has not been around long enough for us to know too much about smoker's lung, the first evidence looks serious. We just don't know yet how much cocaine you have to smoke in order to get smoker's lung, nor do we know the long-term consequences of smoker's lung.

Chronic cocaine use also produces numerous effects on the eyes. "Snow lights" is a term used to describe patches or flashes of white light in the field of vision. One person described it as "Dancing patches of white light, flash-like, that kept darting in and out of my vision." People also have trouble focusing their eyes and report hypersensitivity to light. This hypersensitivity seems to come from a condition called mydriasis, in which the pupils stay dilated and cannot close down in response to light, thus making the eyes very sensitive. People who are having trouble focusing their eyes report that they see things fuzzily or have a sensation that there are floating objects in their line of vision, mostly in the corners of their eyes. They sometimes report seeing double (double vision), or perceiving things as bigger or smaller than their actual sizes.

Cocaine is often referred to as an aphrodisiac, having the ability to enhance the sexual experience; yet, over time, chronic cocaine use actually has the opposite effect, causing sexual dysfunction. In men, it reduces sexual desire and impairs the ejaculatory and erectile abilities, so they are either impotent or unable to have an orgasm. Women have their own reactions to cocaine. They often lose the ability to produce vaginal lubrication, making sex uncomfortable and sometimes painful. They report a lot of trouble achieving orgasm and a general reduction in sexual desire. Like men, they ultimately lose interest in sex as cocaine becomes more important than sex (remember the rats?).

Some other less known but common physical effects of cocaine include insensitivity to temperature, both outside and inside the body; changes in body temperature; hyperactivity; tremors; dryness of mouth and throat; dizziness; insomnia; and weight loss. Most cocaine abusers and addicts experience these changes, but do not attribute them to their cocaine use. One woman said, "I thought I was going through an early menopause at thirty-three, I didn't know that my hot flashes were cocaine related; I thought it was my hormones going bonkers. I thought something was weird, but I never thought of the cocaine. . . . "

These are some of the more common physiological effects of chronic cocaine abuse and addiction. Now let's look at a consequence that is less common, but growing in frequency: death. We always seem to hear about famous people dying from drug overdoses, but the papers don't do stories about people out there who are just having some fun on a Saturday night. Maybe because we don't hear about it, we don't think it happens; but it does. It happens every day, in all areas of this country.

According to the medical examiners surveyed through the Drug Abuse Warning Network (DAWN), there was a 600 percent increase in cocaine-related deaths between 1970 and 1980. DAWN/CODAP reports a three-fold increase in cocaine-related emergencies in hospital emergency rooms from 1976 to 1981. During that time period and up until today, there has been an enormous increase in the amount of cocaine smuggled into this country and a concomittent and an alarming increase in cocaine use, abuse, and addiction; therefore the mortality rate is constantly increasing. Treatment facilities are seeing an increase in cocaine-related admissions; the National Institute on Drug Abuse (NIDA) reports a five-fold increase in admissions from 1975 to 1980 (Seidler, 1982). At the Haight Ashbury Free Medical Clinical Detoxification Project, Dr. Darryl Inaba reports an increase from 1 percent to 25 percent of clients coming into treatment for cocaine between 1981 and 1983. On August 3, 1983, the *San Francisco Chronicle* reported on page 1 that deaths from cocaine overdoses may well have exceeded deaths from heroin overdoses in any major city in 1983. At that time San Francisco was no exception—the coroner's office reported that cocaine was appearing more often than heroin in drug overdoses.

The average amount of cocaine that will cause an overdose seems to be 1.2 grams taken intravenously; but much smaller amounts have caused acute toxicity, poisoning, and even death. Death is caused by cardiac complications or respiratory failure. A person who experiences an acute cocaine overdose can die in as little as five to fifteen minutes. So prompt medical care is essential.

The phases a person goes through during an acute overdose begin with a general confusion about where they are and what is happening around them; they report feeling dizzy and confused. The first physiological signs are hyperpyrexia (an abnormally high fever), followed quickly by clonic-tonic convulsions (where a person's muscles rapidly contract and relax). At this point it is imperative to get medical assistance quickly, because chances for survival diminish the longer the acute reaction goes untreated.

Along with the convulsions, the person's breathing rate could increase while the respiratory system would be diminished; this produces faster but more and more shallow breathing, which in turn may lead to heart arrythmias (irregular heartbeats); the person can die as a result of cardiac complications, respiratory depression, or a combination of the two. In slang terms, when somebody's breathing "bottoms out" and is so depressed that it can no longer sustain life, that is known as the Casey Jones reaction; and it can take as little as five to ten minutes from the point at which a person first begins to feel confused to the moment of death. The only hope for saving a person in this state is to apply life support systems to sustain him or her through the toxic reaction until the body metabolizes the cocaine and flushes it through the system.

Sometimes acute cocaine poisoning has a slightly different appearance. The person may seem very anxious, restless, irritable, confused, and annoyingly talkative. The person may also experience abdominal pain, nausea, and vomiting. At this point, friends around such a person may not know how serious the problem could be, because these early symptoms are fairly common among cocaine abusers and addicts. Cocaine can trigger the vomiting reflex, so this person may be accustomed to vomiting during a cocaine run. As one of my clients said, "Oh yeah, I used to do that all the time. I'd be up all night snorting with friends; my girlfriend and I used to take turns in the bathroom, but she vomited more often than me . . . it was a big joke—'Oh there she is vomiting again. Don't worry, she'll catch up when she gets out; just pass the mirror.' . . . " Thus friends may not recognize the beginning stages of acute cocaine poisoning. What follows in this case is a rapid deterioration of the person's physiological and basic life support systems. The person's heart rate will increase rapidly and breathing will become irregular. If the cocaine poisoning is not reversed quickly through medical means, convulsions and coma can result. The only way to save a person's life in this situation is through hospitalization. The heart and respiratory systems must be stabilized, and sedatives or antipsychotic drugs may be given as needed. If these emergency procedures are not available, the person will die from cardiac or respiratory arrest.

We have just seen how cocaine can affect the physiological system, and ultimately, in the most serious cases, how it can cause death. Now we are going to look at how it affects the emotional/psychological system. In order to better understand this, we will first review the physiological bases for emotional changes—because the psychological effects of cocaine are often caused by physiological changes. We started this chapter by saying that cocaine works directly on the brain. We will now look at the connections between the effects it has on the brain and how those effects manifest themselves in a person's psychological state.

PSYCHOLOGICAL EFFECTS OF COCAINE

Cocaine prevents the re-uptake of brain amines (the chemicals that the brain uses to transmit messages to the body) from the synaptic cleft (the space in between two nerve cells) back into the nerve cells. In other words, cocaine acts as a block—the nerve cells can send messages out, but they do not get where they are going and cannot be returned. Thus the brain cannot get its messages out clearly or adequately, and the body and emotions respond by going on emotional "tilt." If a person continues to use cocaine and the brain is continually blocked from returning chemicals to the nerve cells so they can be replenished, the result is depleted nerve cells. The chemicals that should be housed in the cells are instead floating around in the spaces between the cells and bringing emotional havoc to a person's system.

Some of these chemicals that are released into the synapsis (the space between the nerve endings of the nerve cells) are norepinephrine, serotonin, and dopamine. Norepinephrine is a hormone that works as a vasoconstrictor (hence the vasoconstrictor qualities of cocaine); serotonin is an organic compound capable of raising the blood pressure; dopamine is a neurotransmitter that is essential to normal nerve activity. Because dopamine is in the general area of the neurons (though floating about, blocked from returning), the neurons (nerve cells) in the ventral tegmentum and nucleus accumbens (midbrain) continue to fire off their signals. These signals stimulate the reward (or pleasure) center of the brain. Such a high firing rate results in euphoria, a feeling of complete well-being. But prolonged activation of dopamine without the needed replenishing process (which cocaine blocks and does not allow to occur) results in dysphoria, a state of unhappiness. According to one school of thought, prolonged activation of dopamine from brain cells is presumed to be the biochemical foundation of schizophrenia. This may explain why cocaine psychosis looks so much like a schizophrenic episode.

Another problem that emerges when dopamine mediates the reward system (when cocaine takes over the reward mechanism by blocking the re-uptake and allowing the pleasure center to function unchecked) is that survival behavior, such as eating and sleeping, is forgotten. The body is not getting the messages it needs to take care of daily business. Lack of sleep and poor nutrition exacerbate any emotional problems a person may be experiencing and further break down the body's ability to cope. Thus emotional reactions are worsened by biochemical reactions, which in turn prevent further messages of survival such as "eat" and "sleep" from getting through the confused brain system. The addict's emotional state see-saws out of control and often escalate into bizarre behavior.

Bizarre behavior falls under the label of cocaine psychosis, which can be divided into three stages, each more serious in severity of symptoms. The three stages do not necessarily follow in a steady progression from first to last; a person can skip around and repeat different stages out of order, or become stuck in one stage for a while.

During stage one the person is depressed, irritable, and restless after doing cocaine. I call this "stimulation overload." It seems to occur when the brain cells are depleted of the basic biochemical neuro-transmitters, as described above. Once these return to the brain cells (after the effects of cocaine have worn off), the symptoms generally wear off, especially if the person eats and sleeps normally. Stage one is the beginning swing of the yo-yo in the euphoria/dysphoria cycle that can be very "crazy-making" in later stages of cocaine psychosis.

Stage two is characterized by even more erratic mood swings and an increasing sense of paranoia. In this stage the addict is aware of the paranoia, begins to feel less in control of moods, and often begins to wonder what is happening to his or her life.

Friends begin to notice changes in such a person's behavior and moods and begin to wonder about the shifts and increasing inconsistencies in behavior. At this stage the addict may begin to miss appointments on a fairly regular basis and to appear more and more depressed, frenetic, agitated, listless, apathetic, or angry with increasing frequency and no apparent reason. These symptoms often confuse people who have known the addict before cocaine use began. If a person at this stage stops using cocaine, the mood swings will level off within a few days to a week.

Stage three is the most severe, the one in which violence has been known to occur. In this stage the erratic mood swings become more noticeable (even those who had wanted to ignore them and pretend that nothing was wrong can no longer ignore them); and the person often withdraws completely from close friends and finally even from fellow cocaine users. The addict appears aggressive, hostile, depressed, agitated, and at odds internally as well as with the world at large. Part of this stance is caused by increasing paranoia and the increasing belief that the paranoia is valid.

At this point the addict has lost perspective on reality and has moved into a paranoid delusional state, which may include visual, auditory, and tactile hallucinations. People in this phase have attacked others whom they believe to be plotting against them. In this case the frenzied addict will attack first, if physically capable of doing so, justifying the attack as self-defense. It is very difficult to convince people in the middle of a cocaine-induced psychotic episode that they are hallucinating; you need a lot of time to get through to them. Negotiations with a person in a psychotic episode must be handled very carefully to prevent a violent outburst.

People have committed suicide while in the middle of a cocaine psychosis because of the certainty that "they are all against me and closing in for the kill," and they'll kill themselves rather than be killed. Those kinds of deaths are so tragic. In most cases, all the person needed was a few days off the drug, some sleep, and some food. Where suicide is a possibility, it may be necessary to give the person a low dose of an anti-psychotic drug for a few days until he or she gets a firm grip on reality again. Cocaine psychosis is reversible if the person is treated in time. Addicts may also commit suicide when the emotional pain they live with on a daily basis becomes too much to handle, and the only way out that they see, in this distorted state, is death. To them, death may seem like a relief.

A milder form of emotional effects of cocaine is called "cocaine blues." This is much more common than cocaine psychosis, although I am beginning to wonder if cocaine blues is really stage one cocaine psychosis. (Luckily, a lot of people get themselves into treatment after experiencing the cocaine blues, so they do not have to experience later stages to see what might have happened.) When users come down from the drug-induced high, they are often depressed, withdrawn, agitated, upset, and dysphoric (a feeling described by some as "nothing seems right," or "everything seems to be in various shades of wrong," or "I would always be aware of how lethargic I felt and how it seemed kind of meaningless without cocaine in my system; that's why I wanted more and that's why I'd get more"). Cocaine produces this cycle of feeling up and down, euphoric and dysphoric, until, over time, those two states blend together into a mushy gray shade of depression, lethargy, and listlessness known as the cocaine blues.

A person who has done enough cocaine to experience the cocaine blues is probably also experiencing a strong craving for the drug when not using it. This craving, labeled "drug hunger," appears in varying degrees of severity from constant conscious haunting images and desire for the drug, to drug-related dreams. People also talk about drug hunger when they perceive images relating to the drug so vividly that they border on tactile and visual hallucinations. These episodes of drug hunger may occur only occasionally, or they may happen every few weeks, days, hours, even minutes. One client I was working with said, "It's not fair; I've given up the drug, but it won't give me up—these urges are getting ridiculous. I wish they'd stop!" As this client suggests, drug hunger is one cocaine-induced effect that does not necessarily disappear when you stop doing the drug—drug hunger often lingers for months and even years.

Another disturbing psychological effect induced by cocaine is the sensation that bugs are crawling under the skin. This probably occurs in late stage two or stage three cocaine psychosis, because it involves a tactile hallucination. Nobody can see the bugs, but addicts feel them so plainly that sometimes they scratch their skin until they have large red welts. In extreme situations, constant scratching produces skin ulcerations and infections that require medical care. Cocaine bugs begin as a minor irritation, and can end up being very emotionally upsetting as the itching spreads throughout a person's whole body with no relief available. (Stopping cocaine use, of course, will stop the bugs; but people usually do not connect the two.) I once saw a woman whose face and hands were covered with bloody, partially healed sores caused by her incessant scratching and trying to get at the imaginary cocaine bugs under her skin. This woman will probably have permanent scars to remind her of her experience.

Now that you are aware of the dangers of cocaine, you may be concerned about someone you know—how can you "save" him or her from a cocaine demise? You can't; the only person who can save the addict is the addict. But there are steps you can take. Those steps include talking, education, expressing your concerns, and, as a last resort, organizing an intervention. We'll take a look at how to do this in the next chapter.

7. An Intervention

An intervention is a meeting in which significant others confront an addict with what they see as very destructive behavior on the addict's part. It is appropriate when the people involved have all unsuccessfully tried, individually and at various times, to "get through" to the person about his or her drug usage. Each of these people has dropped some hints, some concerns, some suggestions to their friend, relative, or work associate, but none of those suggestions and concerns have done anything to change that person's drug-taking behavior. When a few of these significant others truly believe that someone is getting into trouble with cocaine, then it's time to seriously consider an intervention.

This confrontation needs to be based on specific incidents of inappropriate or dangerous behavior on the part of the drug user, which the person doing the confronting believes has been caused by or influenced by drug use. Basically, the significant others supportively confront the addict with the addictive behavior, and the consequences they see (which the addict will deny). The interventionist—a professional, not one of the friends—then presents the addict with some positive alternatives and directions. You may ask, "What right do these people have to make decisions for the addict that drugs have become a serious problem?" Or, "How dare they be so presumptuous?" That is part of the role an interventionist plays: Making sure people involved are not being so "presumptuous." The interventionist gathers data and assesses whether or not the person in question does indeed have a serious drug problem. If the answer is yes, then an intervention, although it may infringe on a person's privacy, may also save a person's life.

Interventionists are professionals who have special training in doing interventions. They may be licensed, degreed, or be paraprofessionals with a lot of experience in the field of chemical dependency. Interventionists make sure people present facts and concerns based on those facts rather than accusations and admonishments. They facilitate group dynamics and act as objective outsiders in what is often an emotionally laden experience for everyone involved. Many inpatient and outpatient drug programs have interventionists on their staff; and many private practitioners specializing in chemical dependency are also available for interventions. The cost varies widely, from free services (if there is a reasonable possibility that the person will enter into a treatment program with the agency where you contracted for an interventionist), to an hourly fee schedule.

When I initially plan an intervention, people frequently express to me their fear of hurting the addict's feelings, or of losing trust and friendship. At times like that I try to deal with each fear separately. I tell them the addict's feelings may be hurt for a while, at being found out, "but they will be hurt a lot more if you don't confront him and he goes on thinking everything is fine so that he continues to make a mess out of his life, or much worse, even dies from an overdose. What are a few temporarily hurt feelings compared to death?"

I use the term "temporarily" hurt feelings, because once in treatment addicts usually forgive the people who did the intervention. After they can clearly see what they have been doing and where they have been headed they really appreciate the efforts by the people who did the intervention.

Concerning loss of friendship: Again, treatment will help; if the person goes into treatment, and cleans up, and begins to see things without a drug-distorted view, friendships will almost always remain intact; in many cases the friendships grow stronger from the caring shown during an intervention. Likewise, loss of trust becomes a moot issue if the addict agrees to go into treatment. Trust is relearned, and it becomes clear that all the people involved in the intervention have had the addict's best interests at heart and intervened because of their own trust. Somehow, even through the drug-hazed foggy perspective, the person somehow heard them and seriously considered the options they presented. When the addict acts on one of those options, the mutual trust is validated. I try to allay people's fears and say something like, "No, an intervention is not a mean thing to do; in fact, it is a very gutsy and caring thing to do. It's not mean at all, what could be mean about trying to save someone's life?"

AN INTERVENTION IN THE HOME

In the most ideal situation for an intervention, a number of significant others have met with the interventionist, talked about what each of them wants to say, planned the logistics, and then one of the people involved gets the identified person to agree to meet with them to talk. That way a stranger is not sprung on the probably already paranoid addict unannounced.

If possible, you want the person to know a little about what's going to be happening. Often that is not possible, because the addict wouldn't show up if he or she knew a number of people were coming over to talk to him. In fact, this only seems to work with people who are already fairly willing and ready, who know their lives are a mess and are desperately hoping someone who has it more together will come in and rescue them. Even these people may initially act hostile and be angry, but that's to be expected; they will usually give up their anger after some support by the interventionist and those there for the intervention.

When I arrive, I introduce myself or am introduced and try to make some comfortable talk as we begin. I ask the addict if he or she knows why we are there. The usual response is something like, "Because they think I'm having trouble with coke, and the only reason I let you all come is so I could prove that I don't have any problems and they should stop worrying." Fine. I'll begin there. Sometimes I'll even let a person with that kind of attitude start out first, by telling what he or she thinks is happening. Then everyone else gets a chance to tell what they think is happening. If the addict begins, then the others have a chance to refute that view of reality with their evidence of the addict's distortions and deletions.

I also make it clear that I am there to make sure that everything is said in a caring way. I don't mean syrupy sweet; a caring statement is sometimes very confrontive and upsetting, but it has to be said with a positive intent. If it is, the message is more likely to get through.

I want to make sure people don't use this forum to be vindictive; they can vent their anger, but they can't take accusatory or vindictive stances. They are there to help this person get into treatment, not to get revenge. Throughout the intervention I will, therefore, have people repeat things or say them in different ways if I think they are being unreasonable in their presentation. When the person being intervened upon starts getting defensive, I explain that, "We are all here for a reason—not to alienate you, but because these people care, and they care enough to take a big risk and confront you. So please hold back on your defensiveness and listen." Those reassurances are very helpful, and the person usually sits back and can listen some more without being defensive.

The addict's arguing time is over for now, and it's time to let in a little bit of reality. It can't hurt any more than the cocaine has been hurting, and we all know that's done a lot of damage, or we wouldn't be there in the first place. Even the addict can admit that as the intervention continues, and usually the person being intervened upon breaks down and starts talking a little bit of reality too. It is scary, but the addict can usually see through the fear enough to believe what people are saying.

Sometimes you do a perfect intervention; everyone says everything just right and you do a great job of facilitating but the person still refuses treatment. He (or she) is going to continue using drugs and is angry as hell and wants you all to leave so he can go cop some coke and really do it up good this time. At times like that you have to assure the people involved in the intervention that they did a great job, but the person is just not ready for help; he is too hell-bent on his active addiction to do anything else but use right now. I try to remind them that "you can bring a horse to water but you can't make him drink." I tell people when we are planning the intervention that there are no guarantees we will be successful; and if we're not, I try to remind them that we knew going in there were no guarantees. It doesn't take the pain and disappointment away, but it helps to be fore-warned and later reminded of the forewarning; then at least the failure doesn't come as such a shock.

Here is an example of a successful intervention in which the identified person agreed to begin a recovery program. This inter-vention involves a thirty-two-year-old man, "John," his mother, his father, and his best friend, "Brad." His parents arrived from the Midwest after receiving a desperate call from their son. He said he needed something, but wasn't sure what, and hoped they could come out. They were very nervous when they called me, and wanted to do "the right thing"—although they really didn't know what that was. They told me that he had been snorting cocaine every day for at least a few months, though they didn't know how much or where he was getting the money; they re-ported he was very thin and acting very nervous and wanted to know what I suggested they do.

I talked to their son John and got a little more information from him. He told me he was doing about a gram a day and had been dealing "some" to help support his habit. I asked about his history with the drug, and he told me he had started using it with a woman he was dating about a year before. When he stopped seeing her he hadn't done any for about six weeks, until he'd met "Cathy," who dealt cocaine for a living, at which time he had an unlimited supply.

Currently, John was a janitor and worked nights in a major corporation. He said that when he'd started doing cocaine he finally had something to talk about with his fellow workers; apparently cocaine use was widespread as a way to keep "the guys" up at night. He was able to begin dealing to them, using Cathy as his connection. Pretty soon he had enough customers to enable him to get his cocaine free. He said he was impressed at how fast he could get business; how it all seemed to make sense at the time. When I asked him about the legality issue, he replied, "I just never thought about it."

This was John's first experience with drugs on this level. After we reviewed his history of drug usage, it was clear that up until his experiences with cocaine he had been a social user: drinking at parties, rarely getting drunk enough to get a hangover, "smoking some weed now and again, nothing too regular." So his cocaine problem had caught him by surprise. I assured him that it caught many people by surprise.

When John called his parents for help, he described feeling quite desperate. He reported that he had been snorting a gram to a gram-and-a-half each day; he was beginning to get paranoid (although Brad said "beginning" was an understatement, because John had been paranoid for a few months); and it was getting so severe that he wouldn't leave the house for days at a time. Sometimes he wouldn't even let Brad in, ignored his knocking at the door, and had even yelled at Brad to go away and leave him alone. Initially, Brad threatened to call John's parents if he didn't stop doing cocaine. When John began to get scared that Brad would carry through on the threat, he decided to call them himself. Luckily, he was fairly ready for something to be different in his life. He just didn't know what to do.

I invited John, Brad, and John's parents to meet in my office and to be prepared for at least a two-hour appointment. I had asked John to stop doing cocaine for at least twelve hours before he came, and to refrain from all other drugs as well; he had said he would try. Monday morning at ten o'clock they all showed up. The mother, "Ellen," was very nervous. She had had no experience with drugs or the drug culture, and had been horrified to find John twenty-five pounds lighter, all jumpy and jittery, and his apartment a mess with an almost empty refrigerator. His dad, "George," was a heavy-set man who was also nervous but hid it with a very rigid stance; he was clearly "the Rock of Gibraltar" for that family. Brad was thin but in shape, a young man who worked out and looked as if he had been in the sun recently. He looked the picture of health compared to John, who was thin to the point of looking gaunt. His coloring was pallid at best, his clothes were clean but crumpled, and I could tell he had made some efforts to "look presentable." He was very fidgety and quite upset when I told him he couldn't smoke in my office.

   From all present, I felt an atmosphere of real concern and a lot of fear—fear about what had happened to John and what was going to happen to him. I wanted both to educate and support all the people there, and at the same time assess John's situation and come up with a treatment plan. I also needed to see if I thought he needed inpatient or outpatient treatment; ultimately, I had to be able to tell them about their options and my suggestions. I could see all this would take a while. But John, though scared, said, "I'm at the end of my rope. Unless I'm going to make a noose I better do something."

Therapist: I want to thank you all for being willing to come. I know this is a hard time for you, and I hope that by the time you leave here today you'll all feel at least a little relieved because you'll see there are some options and ways you can get some relief.

Ellen: Well, we're very glad Brad found out about you. We just didn't know what to do, and you sounded like you knew what you were talking about, so here we are. I'm just worried about our John. Don't worry about me, I have George to take care of me. We are all here for John.

Therapist: That's a lot of concern your mother just expressed for you, John. What do you think is happening here?

John: Well, it seems like I went a little overboard with this cocaine. I was telling my parents last night that they really don't have to worry; now that I realize what's happening—and their coming out has clarified it— I'll be able to deal with it. I've already stopped seeing Cathy and I aim to cut back on the cocaine. I know I should stay away from it for a while, get my life back in order, and then we'll see where it and me are at later on.

Therapist: So you do see that cocaine has to do with the problems you are having?

John: Oh, most definitely.

Therapist: Well that's a beginning. What I'd like to do, since we have all these folks who care about you here, is get their impressions of what they see happening to you. And then I want to hear yours. I also want to tell you all some things about cocaine that you probably don't know. When we all have the same information to work with, we can figure out what to do next. How does that sound?

All: Fine, Okay, Hmmm, Sure.

Therapist: Now John, some of this may be hard to hear because you have not been one hundred percent aware of what you have been doing and how you have been acting for a few months. It's important that you listen as well and as openly as you can, because some important gaps are going to be filled in.

It's also important that you all tell John what you've been seeing and hearing that has concerned you. Tell him as explicitly as possible with as many examples as you can think of. Okay? Who wants to start?

Ellen: Well, John, I could try and start. If I understand the doctor, I'll start by telling you that your father and I have been very worried about you for a long time.

Therapist: Ellen, try to speak only for yourself and let George tell in his own words what he needs to tell John, okay?

Ellen: Oh, I didn't mean to . . . I'm just so flustered about this whole thing and I do so want to do the right thing for him.

Therapist: I understand that, and I'll be here to help with that as much as possible. Go ahead.

Ellen: Well, as I was saying, I don't know what to do anymore. We—no, I noticed a change, oh, about a year ago. You know, when you were so lonely for a long time, and then you met that girl, and that didn't seem right. You just still sounded kind of low when we talked to you on the phone, and then that didn't work out and really, I breathed a sigh of relief because you really didn't sound too happy through that whole time. And then soon after that you started talking about this Cathy gal and you sounded real excited, so I was glad for you. At first. But then, John, I just don't know, call it "mother's intuition" or whatever you will, but our conversations just didn't sit well with me. You always seemed too excited and that just wasn't like you. I've seen you happy, but not that excited all the time; it just wasn't right. Your father thought I was worrying for nothing, but I just didn't know.

Then you started not calling like you usually do; you know: missing a few weeks at a time and not always being very friendly, and that wasn't like you at all. You never treated us like that before.

You started sounding so, so, well, so unpredictable. We just didn't know what to expect when we spoke to you.

John: Oh, Mom. Come on, it wasn't so bad.

Ellen: I wish that was true John, it was, it really was. And being so far away, I really had no idea what was happening, and I certainly didn't think it was this. I mean, my goodness, we don't even have any alcoholism to speak of in this family; John I just didn't know what was going on. You know, you finally talked about liking your job and getting along with the fellows at work better, and I was glad about that. But I did wonder why, after all this time, all of a sudden it was happening. But I was glad for you and I tried to ignore that nagging worry.

Then just about two months ago we called you and you didn't know what we were calling about. You sounded, quite frankly, a little crazy. You were accusing us of not loving you and abandoning you with "all the rest of them." I must say, John, that phone call had us both more than a little worried. Your father even wondered.

And then you started calling at night—well, night there and early morning for us; you said you were calling from work, but you had never done that before. I was afraid you had lost your job. I asked you if everything was all right, and you said yes, but . . . John, and then you started answering us with this high-pitched laugh that sounded just too high-strung for you. I was afraid you were having a nervous breakdown, that's all I could think of. I was ready to come out here, but you kept saying everything was fine and you'd be home at Christmas to prove it. You made it real clear that you didn't want to see us just then, so we tried to respect that.

But John, the phone calls. A couple of times when we called you, you sounded drunk and you got us off the phone just as soon as you could. Now John, in all your years you have never sounded drunk in the morning or the afternoon and we talked to you at different times and you were slurring your speech. I just couldn't even believe it was happening. Your father and I didn't even compare notes on our phone calls at the time, because he couldn't believe it either.

You never even drank much as a teenager, and all the time we were too far away and too naive to suspect . . . [Wiping a tear away] I just wish I had known.

John: Oh Mom, but I didn't want you to know.

Ellen: But why not? We've always been such a close family, we could have helped you. Why did you wait till now, till it's so late?

Therapist: Later, when I tell you more about cocaine, I think you'll understand more why John didn't call you earlier. And I think what you're saying about being such a close family is true, because he did call and you are here and he is listening and you are helping now, and that's more than a lot of families get to do. I would hope you can all spare yourselves the extra pain that can come from asking "why didn't I" and "why didn't you?" and "I should have known." Addiction is an elusive disease, and none of you knew about it; you just didn't have the knowledge to know. And another thing, addiction is so elusive that often even with the knowledge it can still creep up on a person and strike them unawares. So please don't blame yourselves; you can let that one go.

Ellen: Thank you for saying that.

Therapist: You're very welcome. John, do you want to respond to your mom, or do you want to hear what everyone else has to say?

John: Geez, I really don't know what I want right now, besides a cigarette and maybe something to calm me down a little.

Therapist: Something?

John: A Valium would be fine.

Therapist: Not for you, none of those anymore. We'd better talk about how many of those you've been taking so we can figure out if you'll need detoxing from them.

John: Detoxing?

Therapist: Valiums are very addictive, and you can get pretty crazy coming off those things if you have become addicted to them. I know this is hard for you, but hang in there. No Valiums available or allowed here. Let's get back to what your mother was saying, and we'll deal with the Valium later.

John: How do your other patients get along?

Therapist: Don't worry, you're not being singled out here for "no instant relief allowed"; they all learn how to deal with this kind of stuff. Just cause it's hard doesn't mean it's not doable. Let's get back to your mom now.

John: It's hard to hear her say those things. I didn't mean to worry her. It sounds worse than I remember it back then.

Therapist: Tell her and not me. It's important for you to hear what this all sounded like to people who were not under the influence of drugs, because drugs have a tendency to distort your reality and your thinking. You're doing fine.

John: Mom, I don't know what to say yet. I'm still kind of a mess, but I sure am glad you're here.

Ellen: Me too.

Therapist: Okay, who's going to go next?

George: Why don't you, Brad? You've been seeing him in person; I can wait.

Brad: Well, I'm not sure what to say. I'm not really his family. I'm your friend, John, and I've known you a long time, and like she says [pointing to therapist] I guess I'm here because I want to see you back to the way you were. Shit, man, you've been going crazy here for a while, and this has got to change. You just don't listen to anyone anymore, and nothing's important but that cocaine. I'm scared to say some of this in front of your parents, but Dr. Baum said it's best to get it all out so we all know really what we're dealing with. So I'm going to just have to trust that she's right and she knows what she's doing.

John: I really don't want to hurt them.

George: John, this is not about our hurt. This is, as Dr. Baum says, about your life. And given how serious things seem to have gotten, I think we need Brad to tell it all—at least maybe it'll shed some light for your mother and me. Look at yourself, John. You're half your size—what do you weigh? Don't you realize why we're here? It's too late to worry about hurting us.

Brad: Well, as best as I can recall, when John started going with Trish—over a year ago already—that's when he first started doing cocaine. Actually, we both started at about the same time. Only I didn't like it so much, and the expense curtailed my doing it right from the start. Trish knew a lot of people who had it around a lot. So, John, when you were seeing her, you'd tell me about parties you two would go to, and that there was coke there and you enjoyed it. As far as I remember, at that point it was pretty recreational, like drinking and weed had always been. I feel bad saying this now, but at the time I envied you. I did. You were having so much fun, partying, dancing, meeting new people . . . but then you stopped seeing Trish. I never did get that story, but anyway, you were in the pits for a long time. You didn't even want to play tennis with me, and forget raquetball. You just moped around a lot as far as I could see. There wasn't anything I could do . . .

Geez, this is harder than I thought. John, I just don't know, but somehow you've changed, you've changed a lot and I'm scared for you.

Therapist: Brad, I know this is hard, but could you please tell John how you've seen him change and what that's been like watching him over the last year?

Brad: I'll try. . . . It's been horrible! To see your best friend start changing. I mean first it was Trish, at least that sounded more glamorous. But Cathy, she had you fooled from the start. Or maybe you had her fooled. The biggest thing now that I think about it was how your talk changed; everything was all about cocaine. I mean all your stories started revolving around when you got high and did something—that just wasn't like you, and when I tried to point that out you got angry and said I was just jealous. And maybe some of that was true, but after a while I wasn't jealous because I didn't like what it was doing to you.

You started getting so cocky. And when you let it slip out that night that you had started to deal and you were making extra money on the side and could get your coke free, man I knew you were in trouble. John, that just wasn't you.

And you told me I was just being a drag because I tried to get you to look at what would happen if you got busted and if it was all worth the risk—you just didn't want to hear that.

Maybe that was around the time you stopped returning my calls. . . .

John: Oh, come on, Brad. I did so return your calls. What are you talking about?

Brad: No you didn't. You wouldn't call for days; you even hung up on me a few times. And you kept avoiding me. Maybe you don't remember, but I do. Sorry, buddy. I don't have the times marked off on a calendar, but they happened. At first I was pissed at you, but later I started getting scared for you because it was like Dr. Jekyll and Mr. Hyde had taken over. I signed you off for a while because you were being such an asshole. It just wasn't worth it.

Therapist: How was he being an asshole?

Brad: Well, he was, like I say, avoiding me. And when we did meet he'd be hyper as hell, it was hard being around him. Lately he'd be going into the bathroom if we were out someplace, or if we were at his house or my house he'd pull out his cocaine and do it up right there. That's when I knew something was wrong with him. And then he called me when he lost his job. He actually accused me of being in on his getting fired. I couldn't believe it. John, you were sure I had orchestrated the whole thing because I was jealous of you. Hey, I've known you for years, and I had never seen you crazy like that. I don't know if you remember that conversation.

John: Not very well.

Brad: Well, my memory may be a bit hazy from the shock, but I tried to reason with you and you were just not going to buy it. You had this conspiracy thing going and you were not going to give it up. You finally hung up on me, saying I was being unreasonable and you weren't going to put up with my shit anymore, and besides you weren't interested in listening to someone who would frame you like that. Do you know that you even threatened me? You said that I better not come around, because you might just kick the shit out of me, and if I ever did anything like that again I better watch out. You were totally nuts on the phone that day.

John: [With his head in his hand] But I thought . . . I just didn't know . . . Shit, now what? This is getting to be too much. Really, come on, I've heard enough. [He puts his head up and his eyes dart around the room] I'd really like to leave now and finish up another time. I gotta go.

Therapist: Say, John! [John reaches for his coat; Mom and Dad are half out of their seats] John, hold on a second there if you can. Okay. You want to come back another day and finish up, huh?

John: Yeah.

Therapist: Why?

John: Why? Are you crazy too? Why not? You think I need to hear all this shit? Wait, yeah you do, but do you think I want to hear all this shit? The answer, lady, is no. N-O! Understand?

Therapist: Yeah, I think I do. And I also think that a part of you, the part that called your parents and asked them to come out here, also wants to hear all this. And that part needs to hear all this. John, if you don't get a chance to hear what reality has been like, then you don't get to make a good choice on what reality to choose from here. John, you can do anything you want to do. If you leave my office right now you're closing down some options. You can do that, you really can. But if you do, then what? You'll get some more coke? And then what? You'll have fun? Hey

John, has it really been so much fun lately? If it was, why did you call your folks? Why did you agree to come in here?

John: I called them because I didn't want Brad to, and I came in here because I was under the mistaken assumption that you could help. But if help to you is this crucifixion in front of them [he points to his parents], you've got another think coming.

Ellen: Oh, John, you've got it all wrong.

John: No I don't, Mom; you've just been taken in by her. How do you know this is the right thing to be doing?

Ellen: I don't know that for sure, you're right. But I'm willing to go through this and see what she has to offer. John, this is only the beginning, and you're clearly so upset. Let us try to help you.

Therapist: Are you willing to sit back down again even if you really do want to leave?

John: Oh, shit! What the hell do I do now? Look, I don't like hearing all this stuff.

Therapist: Why not?

John: Are you crazy?

Therapist: That's the second time you've asked me that. No, I'm not crazy, and actually I don't think you are either. I think you've done some pretty crazy things in the last few months, but I think that's all from doing too much cocaine. . . . Did you know that too much cocaine makes you crazy?

John: Huh?

Therapist: You know, everyone thinks it's a "fun" drug, but it's really very dangerous. It makes people have incredible mood swings, up and down, lethargic and listless and frenetic as hell; then it makes you paranoid, like when you accused Brad. That wasn't you accusing Brad, it was you under the influence of cocaine, just like I don't think all of you wants to leave here right now, I think the active addict in you wants to leave so we don't help you get healthy again, because that's threatening as hell to the newborn and strong addict in you; but your survivor is willing to stay and listen. And, at least for now, that part has won out.

John: I didn't know all that.

Therapist: Most people don't know all that, and there's lots more to tell you. Can we give your dad a chance and then I'll tell you some more little-known but important facts about cocaine?

John: Yeah, and sorry for . . .

Therapist: Think nothing of it. I'm just glad you're still here. Thanks for that and for the apology.

George: I guess it's my turn. I'm a little surprised at what I've heard today. I don't have any experience with drugs myself, and I was always proud of John for not getting involved when he was a teenager and that was what a lot of kids he knew were doing. I guess I never told you that, John, but I was thankful. I think I attributed that to how you were brought up. Your mother and I never indulged, so I assumed you had learned from us. And maybe that's why I'm so surprised with this happening now. Why now? If you were unhappy in your job you could have found something else. I just don't understand.

Therapist: George, the way you brought up John has nothing to do with him getting into trouble with cocaine.

Cocaine is a very powerful drug. It's been known since the turn of the century that cocaine is the most psychologically addictive drug known to mankind, and right now America is hosting a cocaine epidemic. Yet its users just do not know how dangerous the drug is. When John started using it he thought it was like liquor or marijuana—that he could use it sometimes and not have any problems with it. He did not know it was much more seductive and addictive. Please don't blame yourself. You didn't cause John's addiction.

George: John's addiction? What do you mean? Is John an addict? He just got into a little trouble. Surely with a little will power he'll be able to stop, now that he sees where it's gotten him. Won't you John? You just need some sleep. We'll stay out here for a week and Mom can cook you some good meals, get some fat on your bones, and by the time we leave you'll be well on your way back to normal. Right, John?

Therapist: John?

John: Dad, I don't know if it's that easy. You see, I tried to stop doing cocaine already. And even to get here today—she asked me not to do any for at least twelve hours before coming in here, and I thought I could; I didn't think there would be any problem, but I did do a little bit this morning. Just a little, not as much as normal, but when I woke up I couldn't face this without it. So maybe she's right, maybe I am an addict.

George: I don't like to hear that.

John: Neither do I.

Therapist: You know, I think a lot of our stereotypes about addiction make that a very scary term. Addiction is a disease. And if you have it, you need to get treatment. It is a chronic, relapsable disease that can be fatal if you don't get treatment. But with treatment you can live a very good life. In fact, the quality of your life can be better than before.

John: Oh yeah? I want to hear more about that.

Therapist: Okay, I'll tell you more, but first let's have your dad give us his impressions. He started, and then we got sidetracked. Let's get back to him.

George: I'm not sure what to say, John. . . . Your mother started pointing out the differences after we spoke to you on the phone, and at first I thought she was being overly concerned. But then I started seeing what she meant. You started sounding like you were out of breath, like things in your life were moving too fast for you. I wondered about that, but at first I thought maybe you were just having some fun. But when the calls started coming early in the morning and in the afternoon, and you were actually slurring your words a few times . . . That was just not like you. You never were a drinker, not like that.

It seemed kind of fishy when you called when you should have been at work. I didn't quite understand that. And you started being so short with your mother and me on the phone. It seemed that as soon as you heard it was us, you wanted to get off as soon as you could. You used to like to talk to us.

And then—I better bring this up now. Ellen, I didn't tell you about it because I thought it would upset you, but I have to tell you John, that when you called me at work a couple of weeks ago and asked for that loan—well, I just knew then you were in some kind of trouble. I only hoped it would blow over. Now I sent you some money, but not all that you asked for. It was just such a cockamamie story you told me, about wrecking a friend's car and needing to get it repaired and it would cost $2,000. John, first of all, where was your car? Where were your savings? You always have a savings account; since you've been little you have been proud of having a growing savings account. Now that I know, I'm glad I didn't send you the full amount. I didn't ever dream it was for drugs. You should have known better than to call me.

John: [Looking upset] I know, I'm sorry, only. . . .

Therapist: George, that's another symptom of the disease—John calling you for money and John needing money at all, given what you say is a lifetime pattern of saving. When you are an addict there are no controls over your drug usage. An addict uses uncontrollably, and in the face of negative consequences. Hopefully, now that John knows he has a disease, we can set him up in a recovery program that will work for him. John's addiction had made it "all right" to go through all his savings, and that's crazy addictive thinking.

George: It sure is. Now what do you mean by a "recovery program"? Are you going to send John to some Raleigh Hills–type hospital?

Therapist: I'm not going to "send" John anywhere. I'm going to give him some options, and we'll see where we go from here. How are you all doing at this point?

Ellen: I'm glad you're here, I wouldn't know what to do with all that I'm hearing. I'm kind of in shock, but I want to do what's best for John.

Therapist: Brad?

Brad: I'm relieved and wondering what you're going to

suggest. I'm real glad John's parents are here and I hope, John, you understand we're doing this for your own good. You sure look like hell right now.

John: [Sitting with his head in his hands and hunched over his seat] This is all so hard for me. I feel like I really blew it. I've let you all down and I feel so weak, so worthless . . .

Ellen: Oh, John, please, we don't feel like you let us down. If anything, we let you down—by not knowing and doing something for you sooner.

Therapist: You know something? None of you let anyone else in this room down. None of you had the facts, and one of the things that addicts get real good at real quickly is keeping the facts from themselves and everyone else around them.

Brad, as soon as you realized John was in big trouble you went for help. John, as soon as you realized, by Brad's threat and your own deductions, you were in trouble, you called your parents. And Ellen and George, you were far away and had no way of knowing what was happening out here. You knew something was wrong, but from your son's history you had no way of knowing what that "something" was. And as soon as he called for help, you came out here. So you all did whatever you could as soon as you could. Rather than beating yourselves up for not knowing or doing something sooner, you should all pat yourselves on the back for being as sensitive as you have been and for knowing to call someone in as soon as you did know of someone who knew more about John's problem than you.

Now, where do we go from here?

John: I gotta get off this stuff.

Therapist: I know you do. *How* is the question. You could go into an inpatient program for thirty days. They range in price from $5,600 to $12,000. I know that sounds expensive, but if you have insurance it will often cover most or all of that expense. I have sent a few people to in-patient programs and they have all done beautifully. I like programs that have a strong family program, and when significant others are around they get to participate and learn how to adjust themselves to the effects of the disease. There are also lifetime aftercare groups you can participate in.

John: Forget it, I don't have health insurance anymore.

George: Now, John, don't be so hasty; your mother and I can help, and we want to do the best thing for you.

Therapist: Inpatient care is a great luxury if you can afford it. I have also worked with people with problems like yours on an outpatient basis.

John: What does that entail?

Therapist: You would come in here and see me, probably twice a week for a while, at least a few weeks and probably a few months. We would, together, set up a schedule to fill your time with healthy activities such as eating right and exercising and looking for work and going to meetings. That way we would maximize your chances of not using. You would be too busy. I have learned over time that in order to stay clean you have to spend at least as much time staying clean as you had been spending getting high. By that I mean getting the drug, doing the drug, and coming down from being high. And it sounds like you've been spending most of your time in one or the other of those activities, so we've got to keep you pretty busy with other things.

John: I guess. What are the meetings you mentioned?

Therapist: Narcotics Anonymous, Alcoholics Anonymous, or Cocaine Anonymous.

George: He doesn't have to do that, does he?

Therapist: It's the only known form of recovery that has helped millions of people stay clean. What's your objection to it? You sounded upset when you asked me if he had to go to those meetings?

George: Well, he's not an alkie or anything?

Therapist: I know this is hard for you to hear, but your son is an addict. He is still your son John, but he has a disease, and AA, NA, and CA have been helpful to lots of people just like John. I used to have some very negative stereotypes about AA too, but that was before I had been to any meetings, before I had known anything about the program. It's actually quite nice to go to some meetings. Maybe while you're here you could go to a few with John.

George: Well, I don't know . . .

Therapist: Most of the in-patient treatment programs run on an AA model and have meetings as part of their program. George, it's okay that you don't know, but John, it's going to be essential to your recovery that you give it a good chance. Actually, while John is going to his meetings all of you could be going to some Al-Anon meetings. That is the organization that is geared towards the family members and friends of an alcoholic or addict. It will help you in your own recovery and dealing with this disease. They say addiction is a family disease, and I think all of you have already felt some of its crazy effects. Like trying to second-guess John for the past few months; like you, George, not wanting your son to be "one of those." You all could use some help too.

So, what does this all sound like?

Brad: Boy, John, I didn't realize you'd have to do so much. Maybe you should consider the hospital where you'd be away for a month and get a big start on all this.

Therapist: That is one way of looking at it; however, when he gets out he still has to go to meetings and learn to live in the real world, only now with a drug-free lifestyle.

John: No drugs at all? Not even a little **reefer** now and again?

Therapist: No, not even a little reefer and not even a glass of wine or beer.

John: Why not?

Therapist: When you are an addict, any drug can act as a trigger to your drug of choice. So in order to maximize your chances of staying away from cocaine, you have to give up all drugs.

Ellen: That does sound a little extreme. Surely after a time he'll have gotten back some of his old control.

Therapist: I'm glad you said that, because that's one of the common misconceptions about this disease. It's not a matter of control. The disease has to do with a biochemical imbalance in his system that's been touched off, and he does not have the ability to go back to social drug use of any kind. And that's not because he is weak-willed; it's because he has a disease that he will always have. It doesn't go away.

Ellen: [Wringing her hands] Oh, this all sounds so serious.

Therapist: It is serious. But this is one of those dark clouds that can have a silver lining if John follows a sound recovery program. I've worked with a lot of people like John and have seen them turn their lives around. It can be very exciting. I want to give you all some literature to read so you see what other people say about this. I'll be available for further questions by phone or in person. I know this is a lot of information to take in at once. Please feel okay about asking as many questions as you want now, and later as you think about them.

John: Look, I appreciate you wanting me to check out the hospital programs. But as far as I'm concerned, that option is out. I don't want to take that kind of money from my parents. So I have to do outpatient. Maybe if I don't make it out here, maybe then I'll have to go inside, but I want to try to do it on my own.

Therapist: That sounds reasonable. Are you willing to go to meetings?

John: How often?

Therapist: At first I want you doing something for your sobriety at least once a day. So if you come in here twice a week, then you'll need to go to meetings five times a week.

John: That's a lot to ask.

Therapist: You're right. But we're talking about your life, remember that.

John: I'll try.

Therapist: You're going to have to make a committment, because otherwise you'll be throwing your money away on me . . . I can't help you without the help of the meetings.

John: Let's give it a whirl. What do I have to lose?

Therapist: Your life.

John: It's that serious?

Therapist: John, look at yourself. You have been starving your-
            self to death. If you continue to do cocaine you will
            get sick from malnutrition. And maybe you don't
            know it, but you can die from a cocaine overdose.
            People have died from cocaine that is cut with too
            much lidocaine—it shuts down your respiratory sys-
            tem so you can't breathe, and you suffocate. People
            have died from heart attacks and convulsions. It is
            very possible to die from cocaine. So yes, I do think
            with you and your history that your recovery is a
            very serious matter.

            You have just heard what people who love you
            have said has been happening to you. You're getting
            paranoid, you're getting frenetic, you have uncon-
            trollable mood swings—that's all cocaine related. How
            much more evidence do you need?

John: Enough, enough, I see what you mean. I'll go to the
            damn meetings. I'll try, really I will. And thanks for
            today. It's been hard, but . . .

Therapist: You've been great. How are the rest of you?

Brad: Feeling a little better, not so much like the betrayer.
            Do you really think we should go to Al-Anon?

Therapist: I think it would be helpful. Let me give you all a
            schedule. Ellen and George, how long are you going
            to stay here in San Francisco?

Ellen: Through the weekend, and then George has to go
            back for business. But maybe I'll stay on and help
            John get started again. What do you think, John?

John: That sounds okay, Mom. But I don't know how I'll feel by tomorrow, let alone the weekend.

Therapist: Ellen, if you and George can wait on your plans, let's take it one day at a time. John's right when he says he doesn't know what he'll want by the weekend. He's just going to be beginning to feel again by then, and right now his perceptions are still being distorted from all the drugs in his system. So he'll need a few more days to clear all that out. He needs to stay away from drugs, go to meetings, and come here. Most of all he has to take it one day at a time and, just for today, do no more drugs. Then he has to start tomorrow saying he won't do any drugs that day, and each day like that. Hopefully, on the weekend he'll know if he wants you to stay. And if you do stay, know you're doing it for you and not for John; he has his own work to do. Only John can keep John straight. You can be supportive, but you can't do it for him.

Ellen: I guess I do have a tendency to try to rescue, don't I?

Therapist: It comes naturally with some of us, and we have to watch that because if we rescue too much then they don't learn how to do it alone, and then when we're not there . . . George, how are you doing?

George: Fine, really, just fine. I was doing fine when we walked in, and I'm okay now too. I'm interested to see what happens to John this week, and then after we leave. I just hope . . .

Therapist: We'll all be hoping. . . . Brad, anything else?

Brad: No, not really. Hey, John, you know where I am. As soon as you're ready for some tennis, let's play.

Therapist: Good. Well, I want to thank you all for being here. I know this was not the easiest morning of your lives, but it may have been one of the most productive. I think John has a good chance of making it, and I know he'll have a good support system in all you folks. Again, I am available if I can be of any help. John, let's set up some appointments and then you can all go out and get a good lunch.

Ellen: Thank you so much. I don't know what we would have done without you.

Therapist: You are very welcome. I'm glad I could be here. It was good meeting you.

Brad: My friend was right about you, you do know your stuff.

Therapist: Why, thanks.

George: Umm, I sure want to thank you. Now, about the bill for today. Just let me know, here's my card.

Therapist: I usually have people pay as they go, it's easier that way. John, how do you want to do this? You had mentioned earlier not wanting to take money from your parents.

John: Well, I hate to say it, but I am broke right now. So Dad, if you would pay it, I sure would appreciate that. But please, I'm going to keep track of this because I want to pay you back. This all has got to be a loan just till I get on my feet again, then I'm going to start paying you back.

Therapist: That sounds good. What about you, George? Are you okay with that?

George: Sure, sure, whatever you think is best.

Therapist: Fine. Okay, when can you come in this week, John?

John: I'm unemployed; you suggest the times.

Therapist: Let's meet on Tuesday and Thursday so we can get
            you started right away. How's 2 P.M. on Tuesday and
            3:30 on Thursday?

John: That sounds good. Should my parents come too?

Therapist: Let's have tomorrow by ourselves, and then Ellen and
            George, you are welcome to come back on Thursday.
            Why don't you try to read those booklets I gave you
            so you can ask me any questions you might have on
            Thursday?

Ellen: Fine, we'll be here.

Therapist: I think it's lunch time for you folks now. See you all
            soon.

            [They all leave, saying goodbye and shaking hands]

WHAT HAPPENED DURING THIS INTERVENTION?

John has a strong support system of people who are anxious to
help in any way they can. His father, George, is a rather strong
character; he was frightened at what had happened in his son's
life—a very common reaction. He needed to be educated about
addiction so it would become more familiar and thereby less
frightening to him. He read the literature and had plenty of
questions to ask at the next session.

His mother was very involved in George's and John's lives. She
sees things through "we" eyes more easily than through her own.
After my initial comment to her, since I wouldn't be seeing her
on a regular basis I decided against trying to change her way of
communicating. I was afraid that if I stressed it too much I would
lose her spontaneity and involvement. She would be concentrating
on the way she was speaking rather than just giving her impressions, and John needed to hear her spontaneous account of his

behavior. Besides, he was probably used to the way his mother talks.

Brad was an important local resource for John. He gives the impression that as long as John was in there dealing with his disease, Brad, would be right there with him. He was anxious to have his friend back, and was willing to consider going to Al-Anon meetings.

In the first individual session I had with John, I made sure we had an agreement about his recovery program. We finalized that for the meantime, (we would modify it as we went along) and talked about what we would do if the recovery program didn't work. I wanted to specify what would happen if he started using again and under what conditions we would consider inpatient care. John himself was quite motivated, and a well-designed outpatient recovery program may work for him.

On Thursday, at the family session, I addressed all their questions and told them how they could best help themselves and each other. I stressed the importance of Al-Anon to Ellen and George, and hoped they would be convinced enough to give it a try. I also talked about the disease of addiction as a family disease, and what implications that had for them. This family was very involved and sensitive to each other; if they keep denial at bay, they should do fine.

AN INTERVENTION IN THE WORKPLACE

Sometimes it is appropriate for fellow employees (including a supervisor) to do an intervention. In this example, I was called to a medium-sized computer-related company with about five hundred employees to do an intervention with one of the junior managers.

The supervisor called me to arrange an appointment for a consultation; he was concerned about "Sheila," a junior manager in charge of the night crew. He said she was having some "problems." The problems included money missing from petty cash in larger and larger quantities; being stoned on the job; having been seen buying drugs from one of her supervisees; beginning to come to work late; and generally having a lowered job performance. Sheila had been with the company for seven years and her supervisor wanted to give her a chance, but he didn't know what to do.

After meeting with the supervisor, "Tod," and hearing what he had to say in detail, I asked him if he would be willing to join me in confronting Sheila about her problems, which seemed to fit under the umbrella of "drug abuse"—they were all signs of addiction. I also asked him if there were any other employees who were close to Sheila, and who might be willing to sit down with us and talk to her. Tod said he thought so, and he'd get back to me.

About two days later Tod called and said there were five other employees who were willing to talk to Sheila. That kind of response would be helpful. Tod and I talked some more about the intervention, and we scheduled a meeting for that Friday afternoon. In the meantime, he was going to talk to the people who volunteered and tell them more about what an intervention entailed.

I wanted an hour or so to explain to the participants what would be happening, and go over what they each wanted to say and how to best say it. Then Sheila would arrive and we would talk with her. It would be up to me to assess whether she needed an inpatient treatment program or an outpatient program; Tod was willing to go along with my recommendation. We had decided not to tell Sheila I was coming, and to present the Friday meeting to her as a special staff meeting to iron out some problems—which, in essence, it was going to do. The people involved were afraid that if she knew an outsider was going to be there she wouldn't show up; she had been getting a little paranoid lately, and they really wanted her to come.

On Friday morning Tod called me and said two of the employees had backed out, they were "afraid to hurt Sheila." I understood that reaction; a lot of people are afraid that interventions will hurt people. But in fact, when someone is in bad enough shape to need an intervention, it usually hurts them more to continue to ignore their drug-taking behavior and its consequences. (In this situation the expression "killing him with kindness" has a harsh, cold reality.) I reassured Tod that I could do it with the remaining three employees and himself, so the meeting was still on.

I arrived there at 1:45 P.M. and started the meeting with the three employees and Tod. They all needed reassurances that they were doing the right thing. I told them that we were hoping to impress upon Sheila the severity of her drug problem, and that only numbers of caring people and a supportive confrontation with reality could possibly cut through the denial she had so carefully constructed while she was abusing drugs.

We discussed how to tell Sheila about specific instances that they had seen—her drug purchases; the increasing sum of missing money (that only Sheila could have had access to); her recent lateness and lackadaisical attitude; and, more recently, her paranoia and increased nervousness on the job. One person mentioned that Sheila made frequent trips to the bathroom, and that at a staff meeting she had actually nodded out part way through and almost fallen off her chair. I told that person to be sure to tell that one.

I also alerted them to tell her how they had felt while this was happening. They might say, "I was upset because I like you so much, and when I realized that you had to be responsible for the missing money, I just didn't want to believe it." I told them I was there to make sure we could, if at all possible, get through Sheila's denial and make sure the process was supportive. They all seemed to feel better about what they were going to do, although they were still nervous as 3:00 approached.

At 3:07 Sheila walked in, apologized for being late—"the buses, you know"—and sat down. She didn't even seem to notice or care that a stranger was in the room. She sat with her head bowed.

Tod thanked Sheila for coming. He told her that there had been some problems around work that seemed to be getting more and more serious, and this meeting was to deal with them head-on so we could alleviate the situation. He introduced me and said I was going to help run the meeting and help everyone be able to say what they needed to say.

I thanked everyone for coming and said that I knew this was hard for everyone involved. I turned to Sheila and said:

Therapist: Everybody here is concerned about you. Yes, there are problems around here. And these people, as well as some others that couldn't make it today, are very concerned about some things they see happening with you. I'm going to ask you to hear them out, and then we need to decide what to do with all they are going to be saying. Do you understand?

Sheila: Sure, you're going to blame the mess around here on me.

Therapist: It's not that simple, you may feel like that now, but I hope you won't feel that way at the end of this meeting. Sheila, everyone in this room really cares about you, or they wouldn't be here. They are scared too, but they think you need some help. They're here to give you support and encouragement, not blame. I think you need to hear what they have to say, because it sounds like your perceptions are not as clear as they could be and I think we need their help.

[At this point Sheila is sitting with her elbows on the desk next to her, and her head is resting in her hands]

Therapist: Sheila, can you listen from that position?

Sheila: [Looking up through her hands] I'm listening.

Therapist: Thanks. Okay, who can begin?

Each person told a story about what they had seen happening to Sheila, saying that they were quite sure it was the drugs that were making the difference. When Sheila had not been using as much, these things hadn't been happening; but they had seen a gradual deterioration in her job performance the more she used drugs. They were aware that her cocaine use was increasing, and that in the last few months she had even begun to use heroin in order to come down from the cocaine. They laid out the whole picture—how upset they were and how powerless they felt because nobody was noticing or doing anything. When it was Sheila's turn to respond, I gently reiterated that we were there to help her, and hoped she would remember that as she responded to what she had heard.

Sheila: I feel like such a failure. I mean, I feel so caught. What can I say? I'd just like to disappear. I'd just like to go away.

Therapist: That's a pretty understandable response, and that's what the drugs let you do—go away. But we're here to help you not go away anymore.

Sheila: What do you mean?

Therapist: Let's first hear some more specific responses to what people have said.

Sheila: Well, they're right, about everything. I have been doing more and more coke, and I did buy heroin— but only for the last few weeks. I borrowed some money, but I was going to pay it back . . . it's just hard for me. What you say is right. But one reason why some of you know about this is that you party with me, so I don't think that part is fair.

Therapist: That may be true, but it seems that your partying has gone way overboard. Their use may match yours one day, and then they'll be in your seat. But right now I'm interested in you, Sheila, and what we can do to help you. We'll deal with their problems later, let's help you first.

As the discussion went on, it seemed very clear that drugs were part of that business at all times. "Everyone" knew that Silicon Valley was full of drugs; they were available and being used at all times. The company was not ready to deal with the larger drug problem, but at least they were ready to deal with Sheila. It was clear that her drug use was out of control; she was beginning to add heroin to her drug-of-choice menu and beginning to steal. I felt that she was going to need a medical detoxification, because of her dual addiction. It also made sense to take her out of that environment and place her in an inpatient program where she could experience a drug-free month. Then she could go back into her old environment with plenty of supports, including an aftercare group from the hospital-based program, and individual therapy with me. Sheila said she knew she needed something and was willing to try my suggestions.

I drove her straight from the intervention to a hospital-based program (I had alerted them earlier in the day that I might be bringing someone in). On the way, Sheila said she was still in shock, but knew she was doing the right thing. She again expressed some resentment that a couple of the people in on her intervention also used and abused; I told her that I hoped they would give up their denial before it was too late. I sympathized with her and said I could understand her resentment, but reframed it in different words: "However it happened, you're getting the help you need. And if they hadn't been willing to participate, this might not be happening right now."

At the hospital Sheila called her boyfriend, who packed up some clothes for her and brought them over. He was surprised at this turn of events, but was willing to participate in the family program and wanted to help in any way possible. He had no idea of the extent of Sheila's drug use. She had hidden it well, and as a fairly inexperienced user himself, he was naive about possible signs of addiction. He seemed somewhat cautious, but was willing to cooperate and support Sheila and help himself.

Following treatment, Sheila was able to return to her old job. At this time she is still clean and sober and involved in a strong aftercare recovery program, going to two or three meetings a week and individual therapy. She is doing very well and enjoying life. Since her recovery began ten months ago, a few of the people she supervises have realized their own drug problems (including one who participated in Sheila's intervention) and have also sought help and are in recovery programs of their own. Her influence has been indirect; when other people saw how well she was doing, they wanted some of that in their lives. It has been exciting to watch and be involved in this process at various levels. It's nice to see the spread of health rather than active addiction.

THE IMPORTANCE OF AN INTERVENTION

This chapter has presented a couple of situations in which interventions may have saved lives, and certainly saved some people a great deal more pain, denial, and escape. An intervention is a confrontation with reality that can be done in a supportive fashion. The aim is to get the addict to recognize the addiction and do something about it. It can involve relatives, friends, or coworkers. It is important that all present are there to make a positive impression on the addict, to break through the denial and offer some other alternatives, and put those alternatives into action as quickly as possible.

If the person has too much time to decide what course of action to take, the active disease-thinking may take over and justify lots of "good" reasons not to do what's been suggested. That's why I personally drove Sheila straight to the hospital; if I'd let her go home overnight or for the weekend to think about it, we could have lost her again. It had to be done quickly, while she was feeling vulnerable enough to be willing to let other people who seemed to be more clearheaded tell her what to do.

Once I picked up a client in an emergency room of a hospital after he had overdosed on cocaine and heroin. In the morning, when he couldn't even sit up, he had agreed with my recommendation that it was clear that outpatient recovery was not working and he needed an inpatient, structured program. He had said:

"You just take care of it and get me there." By the afternoon, when he could stagger around, his addictive thinking had begun to impose itself again, and he came up with all kinds of excuses not to go into an inpatient program for a month: He had just met a girl and he had to call her; he couldn't leave his job; his cat needed care. All these logistical reasons started becoming blocks rather than easily surmountable hurdles. We finally did get him into an inpatient program, but only after a lot of cajoling and discussion that had been unnecessary in the morning. That's why I say the course of action decided upon should be implemented as quickly as possible. Haste will minimize the strong avoidance and denial reactions that most addicts have honed down to a fine point.

Interventions are difficult for all participants. They have to be honest about what they have been seeing and how they feel, and sometimes that involves confronting their own behavior. But an intervention can save a person's life and be the first step towards improving the quality of that life. When a person is not ready to change, is not ready to give up drugs, an intervention will not work. But more often than not, a well-planned intervention is an effective process that launches the addict into a recovery program. Then the initial nervousness is forgotten or placed in a broader perspective, and all involved agree: "It was worth it."

8. Obstacles to Recovery

Recovery can be difficult for therapists and people seeking help. Both bring their own sets of reasons, beliefs, and prejudices to the process. Some therapists don't like working with addicts because they are so "uncooperative" and "inconsistent." When I ask what they mean by that, I am told: "Well, they'd rather use than get clean"; "It takes so long"; "It's so hard"; "They seem to be getting better and then, out of the blue, they'll binge again"; "I can't seem to get them to analyze the reasons for their drug usage."

All of these statements are true; and the single underlying theme that explains all of these therapists' frustrations is that they are dealing with addiction. Addiction is a very tricky disease. As with any other chronic or terminal disease, recovery is an individual matter, and it may take time to find the right mixture of treatment ingredients that fit each client. Then, to convince the client to participate may be a whole different task.

The ideal outpatient recovery program includes an individual component (one-to-one counseling focused on drug usage and recovery); a group component (Narcotics Anonymous, Alcoholics Anonymous, Cocaine Anonymous, or a therapeutic recovery support group); and couple's counseling or a family therapy component. An additional feature would be for the partner or family member to attend Al-Anon or Nar-Anon meetings for his or her own recovery. The trick is to get the client involved in the program, and addicts are adept at throwing obstacles in their path.

"OH NO. I DON'T WANT MY PARTNER HERE"

The user's partner is both intricately and intimately involved in the user's distorted and warped view of reality. Somewhere along the way, the partner has been sucked into the user's scenario, and this confused state permeates his or her views of the "real world" and the "user's world." The result is often a stifling and paralyzing inertia:

I knew something was off, but I couldn't figure it out. It was like my mind was permanently out of focus after being pulled back and forth, like a tug-of-war game between what he said and what I could see during my more lucid moments. Maybe I didn't let myself see things clearly because it would have meant I'd have had to face some things about my husband and about our relationship that I wasn't ready to face. You know . . . changes are so hard to make.

Partners are vulnerable to the user's view of reality. They honestly want to believe it when the user says, "Oh, honey, don't worry, it'll be okay. I promise, really; it's different this time . . . I just hadn't realized how hurt you were. I'll stop; I really will." Partners have an investment in that reality. They want what their partner is offering, and it sounds so sincere. Often addicts mean what they say as they are saying it. It's just that they are assuming they can control the disease—though shortly they find out, once again, that they can't.

Because most people want their relationships to survive, they'll put up with a lot in an addicted partner. They often do not know that much of the erratic and irresponsible behavior they have tolerated in their addicted partner was related to the addictive disease. Many co-dependents (cos) do not know that addiction is a disease per se, and they can't understand why the user is not "acting right" or treating them better. In fact, active addicts cannot treat anyone any "better" until they understand their own disease and begin a recovery program. The cos need their own recovery program to deal with their own confused feelings.

Guilt and inadequacy are usually the most powerful feelings experienced by the addict's partner. Guilt, because they may be thinking of leaving or have already left; and inadequacy because they couldn't get their partner to stop using drugs.

One of the first things nonaddicted partners learn in their recovery program is that they are not inadequate at all; regardless of what they have done, or how hard they have tried, they wouldn't have been able to get the addict clean. Although the nonaddicted partner can learn how to support the addict's efforts, only the addicted partner has the ability to get clean and sober.

Early in treatment, it's common to encounter clients who do not want their spouses involved in treatment. Often, clients are afraid to tell their partners about their drug problems because they are afraid the spouse will leave. It's also common for clients to refuse to involve their spouses because the partner doesn't know anything about the problem. Sometimes the partner is also using, refuses to acknowledge that use, and therefore refuses to come in; the person in treatment may go along with that denial and not want to "rock the boat." One of my clients—a young woman—told me that her boyfriend was "real straight . . . he only maybe has a glass or two of wine, once in a while." She went on to say:

Look, he's upset because we are always broke, but if he knew I had been snorting coke for the last two years, while we were living together . . . I just don't know what he'd do . . . and I don't want to find out. So, no. I don't care what you say, I'm not going to tell them. Maybe after I've been clean a while, maybe then I'll tell him.

I really push for family involvement if I strongly believe the significant others are so intricately involved that I can't help unless I get them into therapy too. The following is an example of this kind of intricate involvement. This young woman, "Joan," worked for the city, earning $25,000 a year. She lived at home, paid no rent, and her parents bought all her clothes. Yet, when this woman came in for treatment, she was in debt to the tune of $10,000. She made it clear, however, that she did not want to involve her family.

Therapist: It sounds like you want to have your cake and eat it too.

Joan: What do you mean?

Therapist: You say you want to clean up, and yet I'm saying that unless we get your family in here and get them working with us—helping you, by not making it so easy for you to get drugs (by paying for all your essentials)—you probably won't stop.

Joan: Why not?

Therapist: Why should you, with your home situation backing you up? . . . It's hard to give up drugs. You're talking about a nine-year history of abuse. You've used since you were sixteen years old. You're going to have to learn all new ways of coping with life other than using drugs, and you could use your family's support.

Joan: They won't come.

Therapist: Why not?

Joan: My father drinks a lot, at least eight to ten drinks a day . . . I'm afraid he's an alcoholic . . . and he won't admit it, so he won't come. He can't deal with his own problem—why should he deal with mine?

Therapist: You may be right, but let's give it a try. Having another person in your household being an active alcoholic complicates matters. It's easier for you to abuse; after all, it's all you know, you're only carrying on the family tradition. Like father, like daughter.

            Addiction is a family disease, and it sure sounds like your whole family is involved on several levels with this disease.

Joan: But he doesn't know about my use.

Therapist: I don't believe that. He may not know consciously, but what twenty-five-year-old woman still lives at home and has her parents buy her clothes while she makes $25,000 a year? You have nothing to show for your money; it has to be going someplace. Your family is just blinded by denial. And we have to get them in here so they can see and begin to deal with reality.

Joan: I don't know about that . . .

Therapist: Of course you don't. This is scary as hell to you, it'll blow your whole cushy show.

Joan: Oh, come on, it's not so cushy.

Therapist: There goes your denial. What do you mean not so cushy? They pay you to live and do drugs.

Joan: I work.

Therapist: So what? All your money goes to drugs, and you're sitting here telling me about how crazy the drugs are making you feel and how you want to stop but can't. That's because you have a disease, and the treatment your family is giving you is only going to make your disease much worse.

Joan: Do you really think so?

Therapist: Yes. From all you've told me, I'm convinced that your whole family is actively involved in this crazy addictive disease. Try to take a step back and follow me. . . .

In your family, your father is drinking himself to death. You are making yourself paranoid and beginning to experience uncontrollable rages from your cocaine use—to say nothing of your increased alcohol use to try to cut the effects of the cocaine—and your mother "happily" cooks the meals and your younger sister goes about her own business. Do you see that something is very wrong?

Joan: Well, I guess so, but . . .

Therapist: But nothing. Do you want to live a full life?

Joan: Full?

Therapist: You define how you want to live, and if you don't
            want to be feeling more and more of the crazy feel-
            ings you have been feeling from cocaine, you'll get
            your family in here.

Joan: How?

Therapist: Either tell them on your own that you have a problem
            and you need their help and ask them to come in
            here, or I can call them and tell them that we need
            them in here.

Joan: Don't do that.

Therapist: Okay, I won't. I wouldn't do that without a **Release
            of Information** from you anyway. So will you tell
            them?

Joan: I'll think about it.

Therapist: I guess I can't ask for anything more right now. Just
            please hear that I really think we need them if we
            are going to be able to help you.

Unfortunately, Joan missed her next appointment and did not
respond to two messages I left for her at home and one I left at
work. She called about a month later and came in for a second
session. By then she was experiencing violent outbursts when she
snorted coke. She was considering an inpatient program, although her insurance would not cover an inpatient program. I
again presented the idea of Narcotics Anonymous, Alcoholics
Anonymous, Cocaine Anonymous, and parental involvement, and
again explained why each was necessary. She said she'd think
about it and get back to me.

Six weeks later I received a frantic call from her father, "Bill."

She had "spilled the beans" the night before; he was quite upset and wanted to know what he could do. He and I talked on the phone for half an hour and he agreed to come in for one session.

When Bill arrived, I could see classic signs of alcoholism: he was at least thirty pounds overweight, and most of that centered in his stomach. His face was covered with thin red lines; and his neck, face, and hands all sagged from water retention.

I tried to explain about how cocaine affects a person, about cocaine psychosis, and about the disease of addiction. He was not too receptive. He squirmed a lot, and then said:

Bill: I suppose my daughter told you that I'm an alcoholic.

Therapist: She did mention some concerns about your drinking.

Bill: Well, I'm not. I only have two, three drinks a day.

Therapist: Really?

Bill: Yeah, I come home from work and make up a 10-ounce pitcher of martinis, and then me and the wife relax. She only has one and I have two or three.

Therapist: You split the pitcher.

Bill: Yeah, that's what I said.

Therapist: Are you aware that most drinks are 1 ounce? You're finishing off about eight drinks a night.

[That did not win points with this father. He squirmed more, looked uncomfortable and said:]

Bill: But my daughter's not so bad. She hasn't hurt anybody, she's just kicked in a cabinet door and put her fist through a window.

Therapist: But there's no telling where that will lead. And kicking in a door isn't such normal behavior, is it?

Bill: Well, it's not so bad.

Therapist: What would be "so bad"?

Bill: Hurting another person.

Therapist: But she's hurting herself.

Bill: How's that? Oh, well, she might lose her job, but that's only because she's irresponsible.

Therapist: She's irresponsible because of the drug, the disease. That's one of the main symptoms of the disease.

Bill: Naw, she's been irresponsible for years.

Therapist: She's been doing drugs heavily for years.

Bill: Mmm?

Therapist: We're running out of time. Would you consider coming in with your family to help your daughter and help the whole household run a little more smoothly?

Bill: Well . . . I'll speak with the wife and give you a call.

I never did hear from that father or daughter again. Their family was just not ready for change. They were running on denial and were not ready to give it up. Perhaps one day they'll call and come in, and I can only hope it will be before something serious happens, like the daughter committing suicide or overdosing. That family was definitely moving down the self-destruct path—they had so much momentum going that an outsider couldn't stand in their way and stop them. They would have to stop themselves and then take themselves to an outsider.

"I DON'T WANT TO GO TO MEETINGS TOO!"

Initially, clients often do not like the idea of attending Alcoholics Anonymous (AA), Narcotics Anonymous (NA), and Cocaine Anonymous (CA) meetings. Their disinterest usually comes in two forms: (1) a general objection to going because of the "God shit" or the feeling that "I'm not like those people"; and (2) going to one or two meetings and then claiming they don't see any reason to go because of the "spiritual nonsense," the kind of street people they encountered, or because they want to "get clean on my own." I've heard these excuses so often it's hard not to smile, and sometimes I just laugh and point out the absurdities in their thinking.

I explain that the spirituality involved can be anything they want it to be, that they are not expected to adopt a belief system they do not believe in. I suggest that their personal histories have long ago proven that their own thinking and solutions didn't get them what they wanted, so why not try something else? I challenge them to try two or three meetings a week for two months and then tell me what they think. What have they got to lose?

In answer to the statement "I'm not like that," I simply say, "Bullshit, you're an addict, too." I try to show them that the disease gives them a strong common denominator, and that by going to NA or AA, they are participating in a mutual self-help component in their own recovery process.

When clients are completely turned off to the presence of street-type addicts in meetings, I suggest they could try other meetings, but they also should return to the meeting they didn't like, because "There but for the grace of God go you—and besides, you all have the same disease, they are just further along the road than you." Usually, clients discover they don't like street addicts because that image, that reality, is very frightening. They are so scared they will become like that themselves that they don't want to see the possibility up front, in real life. In these cases, facing their fears is very therapeutic, because they then have an image of what they don't want to become and can begin to create a positive image that they do want to emmulate.

I sometimes hear clients say, "Gee, I'd love to go to the meetings you're suggesting, but I'm just too busy." I respond by telling them, "There are meetings throughout the day and evening, so you can arrange your schedule around them." In addition, I tell them that if they are intent on getting cocaine out of their lives, they must put at least as much effort into staying clean as they used to put into coming up with the money, calling their dealer, going and getting the coke, going back home with the coke, doing it up, being high, and coming down. I point out to them that if they had the time to do all that, they can certainly make time for a meeting. Alternatively, I first ask them what their routine for thinking about, getting, and doing coke used to be, and then we put all that into a time frame. I can then tell them that there are meetings all over the city at all different times, and point out to them that they used to spend X number of hours a day getting, doing, and crashing from coke—isn't it worth an hour or an hour and a half a day to stay clean, and therefore alive?

"TOTAL ABSTINENCE, NO BOOZE AT ALL?"

Most people are initially reluctant to accept total abstinence as a goal and a necessity. (Total abstinence will be covered in more detail in the next chapter.) I believe from my own experiences, as well as from the work of hundreds of other professionals in the field, that the best way to assure success in overcoming addiction to the drug of choice is to abstain from *all* drugs, including alcohol.

This step can take time, and I work with clients for a while to help them come to accept this goal. I try to point out their drug-of-choice "slips"—usages—relative to other drug usage. As they come to see their slips are always preceded by alcohol, marijuana, or other drugs, most come around and are willing to abstain. Those who don't abstain generally find some excuse to terminate treatment, and I suppose they are out there abusing again. I long ago gave up my need to save everyone. I am sometimes sad when someone leaves because I know they are in for more hurt, but then I take myself home and deal with what's left of my own "save the world" syndrome.

"OKAY, NOW THAT I'M CLEAN, LET'S TALK ABOUT SOMETHING ELSE"

Clients often try to sidetrack therapists from specific recovery issues with a line like this: "Now look, you and I both know I had a problem with cocaine, but I haven't used in three days and I feel real good. I mean I feel very confident that I'll be okay and what I really need help with now is ___ ." You can fill in the blank. It could be financial problems, a nutsy spouse, a terrible childhood, or a past trauma. It's all meant to show their willingness to work with you and their willingness to accept their addiction and its consequences. It can work as a smokescreen with an inexperienced drug therapist, and can get you off focus and onto a tangential issue. The end result will be a sabotage of the recovery/therapeutic process.

I try to point out to people that it's good they have been drug-free, and since what we are doing seems to be working, let's keep doing it. Thus I validate their progress and keep them focused on their recovery. By doing this I am also staying in control, I'm not getting sucked into their reality. It's very important for the therapist to stay in control, because the client's life is so out of control and unmanageable.

In this example, "Richard" is trying to lead me off my focus on his recovery and onto his girlfriend:

Therapist: What do you mean?

Richard: Well, other than drugs, actually it's my girlfriend.

Therapist: What about her?

Richard: She gives me shit all the time.

Therapist: Shit [laughing], that can get rather smelly.

Richard: Oh, you know what I mean.

Therapist: No, actually I don't. And while you're telling me about it, try to relate it to your drug usage.

Richard: What do you mean?

Therapist: Well, usually when a person is using drugs heavily, being addicted like you are, your behavior changes. You're moody, lots of ups and downs; and that's hard to relate to. So what often happens is the partner—your girlfriend—has to relate to all those changes, and that puts her through all kinds of changes. So she often gets resentful, frustrated, even angry, and then takes it out on you. Now, that's an example of what I mean when I ask you to tell me about the shit your girlfriend gives you and relate it to your drug usage. Go ahead, it's your turn now.

Richard: But I don't want to talk about drugs. I'm bored with it.

Therapist: I understand that. But drugs have been so much a part of your life for so long that you can't talk about your relationship with your girlfriend—or anything else, for that matter—without talking about drugs, because they have been affecting you and your girlfriend for so long.

Richard: Well, but I . . .

Therapist: Hold on, I'm still talking. I suggest you give up being bored with talking about drugs, because we'll be doing that a lot. I want you to get a very solid picture of how strongly they affected you; how the cocaine controlled every aspect of your life. Until you realize the severity on a gut level, you and I will be battling on every front. You won't see the necessity of AA and CA meetings, of couple's counseling, or of remaining completely clean. Our work has just begun, and it's sounding like you're getting kind of cocky. Five days being clean and you have it under control, huh? Don't kid yourself like that, it could be very dangerous.

Richard: Well, but I didn't mean never to talk about it again. I just wanted to set it aside for a while.

Therapist: If I went along with that I'd be doing exactly what you used to do all the time. You said that every once in a while you knew you had to stop doing cocaine, but then you would shove those thoughts aside and go on using, forgetting about the negative effects, right?

Richard: Yeah, but I don't see the connection.

Therapist: I know you don't. After you've been clean and sober for a while, your thinking won't be so distorted and you'll be able to follow conversations and connections like these better. You would focus on the negative aspects of cocaine, and want to stop. Then you'd defocus, shove the negative aspects into the background, and go on using. We know where that'll get you—right back to using. So let's try something new and completely different, like staying focused on the negative aspects of cocaine, and the realities of addiction, okay?

Richard: Okay, I see what you're saying now. That makes sense.

Therapist: All right, now back to you and your girlfriend. Let's start by talking about how she is reacting to you starting a recovery program and not using drugs.

Richard: She says she likes it, but she's scared of how I'll be.

Therapist: That's a pretty natural reaction for her. How do you feel about it?

Richard: About what?

Therapist: Embarking on a recovery program.

Richard: Me?

Therapist: Yeah, you.

Richard: Pretty good, and scared too.

Therapist: Can you talk to her about your feelings, your fears, your hopes?

Richard: I could try.

Therapist: What about bringing her in here?

Richard: That may be a good idea. I've been thinking about it since you suggested it last time, and maybe we could try it.

Therapist: Maybe. Do you want to set up an appointment?

Richard: Well . . . we can set up a tentative one and I'll have to make sure she can make it. I'm pretty sure I know her schedule, but just in case . . .

Therapist: Fair enough.

ADDICTS ARE SCAMMERS

Drug addicts are usually great actors. They have to be to cover their act. They are involved in an illegal activity that also alters their natural state. They have to be able to make everyone involved with them believe that they are who they appear to be and who they themselves, at the time, believe themselves to be. One man said:

I was telling so many lies all the time that even when I *could* tell the truth, I made something up . . . it sounded better . . . like my constant colds. I told the people I work with that I was going skiing on the weekends. I told great tales about that. Skiing would explain missing work on Monday (I was snowed in), or not having any money (it's expensive to ski), and it even explained my constant colds from the cold air and sweating as I skied and took off too many layers. It was a great cover-up. I know how to ski, and I have been to the places I talked about, so I sounded legitimate.

This man's story is what I call a scam. A scam is something done or said in order to cover up what you are actually doing. Another typical scam is claiming your car is about to be repossessed (which may or may not be happening), and getting people to lend you money. In such a case, some of the money might go to the car, but most probably goes for cocaine.

Addicts—because they have been scamming by telling lies, half-truths, and deleting information—are masters at acting. They have to be. It's the only way they can pull off these scams as reality. It is often difficult for the therapist to tell if a person is telling the truth. While I was working at the Haight Ashbury Detoxification Clinic, people would sit two or three feet away from me and swear or implore me to believe that their eyes were not **pinned**, that they hadn't used heroin. At times I was tempted to believe them, because they sounded so sincere; but the evidence to the contrary was overwhelming. I responded by laughing gingerly and saying, "Oh, come on; do I still look that naive?"

Scamming is a reality that drug therapists have to accept. If a woman tells me she has been clean, the only thing I know for sure is that she wants me to believe she has been clean. If I want to know if she's telling the truth, I need details of what she's been doing, how she's been feeling, how her perceptions have changed; and even then I can't be sure. Only a urine analysis or blood test will reveal "scientific proof"; but even those are not too accurate.

A therapist has to develop a "scamming sense," but even the best get scammed at times. I let clients know that I appreciate honesty so I can help them more. I let them know that I am nonjudgmental and will work with them, regardless of what they put out. Above all, it's important not to get personally angry when you've been lied to. The therapist needs to realize that this is how the person copes.

I often congratulate people for being so good that I didn't catch it, and then I point out how much time we wasted by believing and working with a false reality. Oftentimes, if I've wondered if it was a scam, but went along to see, I talk to them about what I had been perceiving. The client is often curious how I knew. Sometimes I tell them; but I keep it to myself when I think the client will take information about my perceptions and go one or two levels deeper with their scams, leaving me completely unable to tell the difference. This latter is especially true when dealing with a **sociopath**, as opposed to a person who is addicted and has picked up some sociopathic-like patterns to cope with the addiction.

Working in the addiction field is a challenge, and there are some blocks to watch out for. But seeing people change their lifestyles, watching them go from a state where life is totally out of control and unmanageable to a place where they learn how to live drug-free lives and cope with life's unmanageabilities—that is so rewarding, so exciting, so gratifying. Therapists who do not want to work with addicts usually do not know much about the addictive disease process. Once they've learned, the work is much more effective, for all involved.

9. The Beginning: A Reawakening

People generally come into treatment in one of two states: crisis or denial. When cocaine addicts are in a state of crisis, it is usually multifaceted—everything has gone wrong. Their finances are low or nonexistent; their personal lives have blown up or disintegrated around them; their work situations are usually in question, at best; and often they are in debt to dealers, friends, and family members. In short, everything is out of control. Often they want the therapist to make it right, to straighten out their messes—and as quickly as possible.

The state of their personal and business lives reflects the nature of their disease. In addition, an addict's drug usage is out of control; it continues in the face of clear indications of negative effects, and it is compulsive behavior. This is usually where I start during the first session.

I try to reassure clients that they have come to the right place. We can work together, but I assure them that I cannot miraculously save them, that I retired my magic wand years ago when I realized that it really didn't work at all.

I try, whenever possible, to see people only if they have been clean for twenty-four hours, although I will sometimes, in a crisis, settle for less. I want to have as much of their minds as possible. If they have been using heavily, even a twelve- to twenty-four-hour respite will not result in a clear mind, though it will be clearer than if they had just used. I also want them to begin to know, on some level, that there is a possibility of not using drugs. At this time I don't verbalize my reasons, but leave it for them to discover later on—I don't want to get them further discouraged before treatment starts if they can't stay clean the required time. The last thing they need is another failure. By the time they see a therapist, they are feeling very badly about themselves and all that they have lost through their drug usage.

Just because a person has made an appointment, and has shown up, doesn't mean he is ready for treatment. He may be flirting with the idea, scared of the idea, or just plain overwhelmed and reaching out for some possible solution. Cocaine addicts and abusers are used to "quick fixer-uppers" and "instant highs." When I begin to talk about a full recovery program and they realize how much time it's going to take, many do not come back; they begin to miss their appointments or cancel all further appointments. I have learned that they are not rejecting me, that I haven't failed; they're just not ready. I call them a few times in the next few months, and often they are ready for treatment at a later date.

Sometimes I set up recovery programs for people and they come to their appointments with me, but won't go to NA or AA, or they slip fairly regularly for awhile. I will continue to see these people if I feel they are in what Paul Ehrlich, of Forest Farms, a residential recovery program in Marin County, labeled "a treatment ready stage." If I feel that they are seriously trying, at their own rate, and admit that they deserve a better life, then I'll stick with them. I need to trust my instincts so I don't feel that I am becoming their co-dependent in a negative sense. I don't want a person to be able to say, "I'm cleaning up my act, I'm going to therapy once a week," and still be using regularly. When I become a rationalization for them to be able to use drugs, I'm a dysfunctional co. If I feel that is happening, then I confront the issue and they are given a deadline to "shit or get off the pot." They either begin a recovery program, or we begin a four-week termination process. At the end of the four weeks they are terminated with the assurance that when they are ready to begin a serious recovery program, they are more than welcome to call me.

People who come in and are still in denial are usually referred by someone else—their employer, their spouse, a friend, or a family member. These people often come in only to please their significant others, not themselves. If you can't get them to admit to their problem, you can forget about hooking the addict into treatment.

I find that addicts still in denial are coming as a kind of con—"Okay honey, I'll go for some help." They have no real intention of cleaning up; their only intention is to get their partner temporarily off their back. These setups are fairly easy to see, because they look too good and feel flat; I confront them head-on because I don't want to be sucked into that kind of crazy system. I have to stay out of a crazy system so I can maintain my objectivity and my control. If you become part of the crazy system, the craziness takes over and you lose control. Then the therapy situation becomes as uncontrollable and unmanageable as the rest of the addict's life.

I often feel like a combination of a director and a cheerleader for the first few weeks or months of treatment—a director because I program their time with healthy, non-drug-related activities; and a cheerleader because I continue to cheer them on, encouraging them through rough times and telling them, "Go on, you can do it!" This method does seem to work, so let's consider it in detail.

In any therapeutic process, the first session is crucial. The client is feeling out the therapist both as a person and for therapeutic style, and is deciding whether or not they will be able to work together. At the same time, the therapist is feeling out the client; listening to the way problems are presented; and probably looking for underlying, unstated problems lurking behind the words, actions, and perceived feelings. It is a time of mutual exploration for trust, compatibility, and direction. Clients are generally nervous and scared in any first session. "Will this person understand? Will this therapist be able to help me? Can I trust this person and say what is really bothering me, or will I look crazy?"

Now, add some extra ingredients. Clients who come to therapy for a so-called "cocaine problem" often have some cocaine or some other drug actively affecting their system. If they have been using heavily, they may be experiencing paranoia from the cocaine's own toxic effects; and that, coupled with normal first-therapeutic-encounter jitters, makes for a rather difficult situation. In addition, most people have not yet admitted, nor possibly even considered, that they are probably addicted to cocaine.

Paranoia may also be exacerbated by the issues of illegality. Cocaine usage, itself, is illegal. But when you discover that a client is working as a janitor, for minimum wage, and doing two grams of cocaine a day (or is in middle management in a corporation, grossing $3,000 a month and using three to five grams a week), the obvious question is, "Where is the money coming from to buy all that coke?" Chances are that you'll be in even more illegal territory. Many people with large cocaine habits deal coke (sometimes in a very limited quantity to good friends so their own coke is free), or do "runs" (transporting coke from one dealer to another a level down in the chain). Another way people finance their habits is by selling their possessions. One person had reduced a fully furnished mansion to one mattress in one room; all other rooms were bare.

It is strange that people who do runs do not consider themselves to be dealers, or to be doing something dangerous, although runners have also been found in car trunks, very dead. Here again, denial and distorted thinking from continual drug use allows them to justify their actions and feel relatively safe.

Okay, back to the office. Here I am, sitting across from a new client, one who is involved in illegal activities, who may very likely be quite jumpy, edgy, irritable, excited, scared, paranoid, and anxious. This client expects me to solve his or her problems—instantly, if not sooner. My goal for the first session, on the other hand, is to establish a rapport, get some information, give the client important and little-known facts about cocaine, introduce the disease concept, and assess whether or not this person is "treatment ready."

To facilitate all of this, I never take notes—there is no evidence of pads, pens, or file cabinets in my office. This seems to put the client somewhat at ease, although only temporarily; because by the end of the first session, the person is reeling from the barrage of new information. That's fine. I want to catch the person off balance, so that information can penetrate the defenses and denial that have been carefully built up over time.

Most of what I tell clients the first day will have to be repeated, because they will "forget it." The "great eraser," (as Dr. Carole Campana of Ramapo College, in Mahwah, New Jersey calls it) invades their minds—often as soon as they take one step out of my office—wiping the slate clean so they can once again be comfortable in their well-defended views of reality.

By the time clients leave my office after that first session, I want to have obtained the following information: How much cocaine they use daily and weekly, how long they have been using, what other drugs they have used in the past, and what other drugs they are currently using. It is important to ask them what they use to soften the crash after a cocaine run. People usually forget about their secondary drug usage, because they see it as self-medication to take the edge off the coke.

It has been my experience that you can usually double what people report as their drug usage to get a more realistic picture. This doubling is necessary, since people tend to minimize their reported drug intake. They do this for one or more reasons: (1) They are so loaded that they honestly lose track of what and how much they are consuming; (2) they want to please you, the therapist, and do not want to freak you out (after all, they see you as their only hope and they want you to like them); (3) they honestly need to believe their usage is not as bad as it really is, (denial again); or (4) they have never kept track, so they give you their best estimate, one that will put them in a fairly good light.

PROVIDING NEEDED INFORMATION

During that first session I want to give them some information about myself as a person and a therapist—particularly about my knowledge or experience with drug abuse—so they can get a sense that I do, indeed, know what I am talking about, that I may be able to call them on their shit, and therefore I just ma$_)$ be able to help them. Remembering that addicts are the best scammers in the world, I make them aware that I know this, that I'm pretty good at telling fact from fiction (even though sometimes I won't be able to distinguish between the two).

Whether I do this directly or indirectly, using a metaphor or a story about another client, depends on the client in the room and what I perceive he or she will be more inclined to "hear" and take to heart. Basically, by saying this I am establishing that I can help them to the extent that they are honest and willing to reveal themselves to me. If they want to come in, lie, and tell stories, I will work with the lies and stories (if I don't see through them), and they'll be throwing their money away.

Sometime during that first session, after I feel there is some rapport developing, I present my belief in the disease model of addiction, the implications for recovery possibilities generally, and for each individual specifically. This is not the most comfortable portion of the fifty-minute session. In fact, clients squirm a lot when I tell them that they will not be in a full recovery program until they realize they must abstain from all drugs or make a commitment to do so. Often, clients argue that their drinking or marijuana smoking or Valium use is under control, that it is only their cocaine use that has gone haywire. I tell them that I understand their present beliefs regarding this; but in time, when they are free of cocaine, they will learn more about the realities of drug abuse.

I go over the addiction model with them. In order to be addicted to the drug, they have to use cocaine compulsively, have no control over their usage, and continue to use it in the face of negative effects. I want to get enough information about the clients' patterns of usage during the initial session to point out to them how their cocaine behavior displays each of these characteristics. If it doesn't, they may be abusers and not addicts. If they are addicts, I am firm about what the conditions will have to be if they are going to recover from this chronic illness.

I present addiction as a terminal disease. I give examples of

STEP OVER THE LINE

, and those I have heard about or read about, and
: died from overdosing on cocaine or using some
:ut so badly they have died. By telling these stories
ng to scare people into quitting; I'm simply pre-
with the facts and realities about cocaine addiction
in particular, and addiction in general. Cocaine addiction is really
no different from heroin addiction or alcoholism, they are all part
of the same problem—chemical dependency; and they are all part
of a chronic disease that, if left untreated, will cause premature
death.

In this first session, I try to assess the degree of drug use and
determine whether it is recreational, abusive, or addictive. The
dividing line between abuse and addiction is hazy; I would rather
err in the direction of addiction, because a person's life may be
at stake. In addition to assessment, education is critical. When
people have the facts about how cocaine is affecting them physically and emotionally, it will be harder to deny the addiction.

My own style is to be supportively confrontive. I use a lot of
humor, yet I am also quite straight about the facts. I try to use
humor in countering a client's denials, so that we don't begin to
argue and lose track of where we are going by getting caught in
a circular defensive argument of "yes, buts."

I also validate the client's position. People who are addicted
and actively using cocaine have all types of excuses and reasons
for their actions, all of which seem totally justified and reasonable
to the addicts. I try to stress that there are some reasons for these
present beliefs; in fact, a number of them are excellent examples
of symptoms of the disease. I say, "I believe that you believe what
you are saying. But if you'll allow yourself a couple of weeks of
not using, you'll be able to reconsider what you're saying from a
different perspective—and you just may see things differently."

I had seen "Steven" for five months individually, and concur-
rently for two months in a recovery group. When we concluded
treatment I strongly urged him to continue his recovery with
Cocaine Anonymous and Alcoholics Anonymous meetings, but
he was quite cocky about his recovery and did not see the neces-

sity. When I ran into him four months later everything was fine, though I was concerned about the frenetic pace of his business and personal life. When I called him two months later, however, he had just left a twenty-eight-day inpatient program. He raved about Cocaine Anonymous and Alcoholics Anonymous, how important they were in treating the disease of addiction, and how he couldn't drink, either. I let him talk for a while, and then interrupted him.

"Excuse me," I said, "didn't I talk to you about not doing any drugs because they acted as triggers?"

"Oh yeah," he said.

"And do you remember me urging you to attend CA and AA meetings?"

"Oh yeah, I guess I forgot," he said.

As it turned out, he had started using cocaine again during that critical five-month period we had talked about. His perspective had changed, and he now believes what he refused to believe eight months ago. If he had listened then, he probably could have saved himself from another crisis and the inpatient hospitalization, but people can only hear what they need to hear when they are ready to hear it. Therapists have to remember about this selective hearing process so they don't experience too much frustration.

AN EXAMPLE

Here is an example of a first session.

Therapist: Come on in.

Francine: Where should I sit?

Therapist: Anywhere is fine.

Francine: Oh . . . [looking around] okay.

Therapist: So, what brings you here today?

Francine: Well, I guess I have a problem with cocaine.

Therapist: Oh yeah? What kind of problem?

Francine: Well, it's bad, it's real bad. I just gotta stop.

Therapist: You snorting, basing, or IVing it?

Francine: Basing. And I tell you, that shit is wicked. Every day on the way home from work, I stop at this local store and pick me up a freebase pipe. Every day I buy one, because after I finish basing I break the thing. I break it so I won't ever do that shit again. But then there I am the next day, buying another pipe . . . it's embarrassing. I gotta stop going in that store. And besides, my boyfriend found out I was strung out on the stuff and he'll kill me if I keep on using.

Therapist: Wait, wait a second. Okay, you go to the store, get a pipe, and then what?

Francine: I go home, call my dealer, go see him, buy me some coke, and then I go straight back home, wash it down, and smoke it up.

Therapist: How much do you do a day?

Francine: 'Bout half a gram. Unless one of my friends turns me on to more. But now they won't do that anymore.

Therapist: Why not?

Francine: Well, the other week, I got so depressed one night I took a bunch of pills. I wanted to just end it all. Every once in a while I get like that. It's all too much . . . you know?

Therapist: Yeah, I sure do. But what's all too much in your life?

Francine: Well, the coke for one. I'm in debt. That's not like me. I always have a savings account. I had $3,500 saved up and it's all gone. And my parents, they even notice a change. They keep saying "What's wrong with you?"

Therapist: What do you say?

Francine: Oh, I say, "Nothing," or "I'm just feeling bad." But they're beginning to look at me kinda funny. See, everyone around me does drugs. There's lots of people in our neighborhood that got strung out on heroin, but I never got in trouble before. I was always the good one. My parents were always proud of me. I don't understand what happened. I don't do heroin, but I can't stop doing this drug. I mean to, but the next day, there I am, back at that same store. I'm not even embarrassed till later.

Therapist: Hold on a minute. You just said you don't understand why you keep finding yourself using it, even though you don't want to, right?

Francine: Yeah.

Therapist: Well, did you know that cocaine is very addictive?

Francine: You mean like heroin?

Therapist: Sort of, but it's different. Heroin is physically addictive, so after you use it a while and then you stop, you go through physical withdrawal symptoms— like chills, sweats, cramps, and you can't sleep. You're also real irritable and moody coming off heroin. But with cocaine, it's different. Cocaine is psychologically addictive, which in some ways is harder to deal with. Remember Richard Pryor's movie where he says, "I was walking down the street and my pipe was calling after me . . . "? It's sneakier. The drug urge just comes up and into your mind, and it's like your mind has no control over your actions and you just go for it.

Francine: Yeah. That's what it's like, but why?

Therapist: It has something to do with a biochemical trigger, and then a biochemical reaction to that trigger in your brain. I'll try to explain it, but it's rather complicated and I'm not sure I even understand it all . . . [I take a pad of paper and draw nerve synapses and show how the natural adrenalin jumps from synapse to synapse and then back again to replenish itself. But cocaine acts as a blocker and the natural adrenalin can't replenish itself] Think of it as two balance scales. When you put cocaine in your system, it puts one of the scales off balance, and then everything is swinging out of control. Basically, I want you to know that it's not your fault. It is not that you don't have will power. It is the drug and the addiction and you don't have control over it.

Francine: What do I do?

Therapist: You've got to admit you don't have control over the drug, instead of trying so hard to stop and then beating yourself up for not being able to. Then you have to give it up. Go for abstinence from cocaine and all other drugs, including alcohol.

Francine: Just like that?

Therapist: Well, not quite. Unfortunately, it's not that easy, but we'll work together and get you there. How long have you been basing every day?

Francine: Only about two and a half months.

Therapist: Good, then at least you haven't been doing it too long. That should make it easier to stop. It's not like you've been doing this for years. And you say everyone around you does it?

Francine: Yeah, my family, my friends, my boyfriend; he does other drugs, too. That's why I thought it was okay. And you say it's addictive?

Therapist: Very. And it sounds like you recently got what we call the disease. Addiction is a disease; when you are using a drug compulsively and you can't stop even though you want to, and when you continue to use even though you know bad things are happening to you, like going in debt, then you have the disease.

Francine: Oh, no.

Therapist: I know it sounds scary, but actually it is treatable. It doesn't have to be lethal, although I know of people dying from cocaine.

Francine: Dying from cocaine?

Therapist: Oh yeah. You can overdose from too much cocaine, or if the stuff it's cut with is bad, or there is too much cut. . . . A friend of mine died a while ago from some cocaine that was cut with too much lidocaine; it shut down his respiratory system so he couldn't breathe.

Francine: I didn't know that.

Therapist: Most people don't, and that's why so many people feel so bad when they want to stop—because they thought they were using a safe recreational drug, and it turns out they aren't.

Francine: I wish I had known, because then I wouldn't be in trouble now.

Therapist: I wish you had known too, but unfortunately, word isn't out on the streets yet.

Francine: Why not?

Therapist: I'm not sure. Maybe it just hasn't been around long enough for people to realize . . . have you ever felt real different than you usually do when you've used coke?

Francine: How do you mean?

Therapist: Irritable, jumpy, paranoid?

Francine: Oh yeah, most of the time now. It didn't used to be like that. It scares me sometimes.

Therapist: What scares you?

Francine: Well, it's kind of funny. Everytime I base now I get scared that the cops are coming. So I keep running to the window. It seems like I take a hit on the pipe, sit back, get nervous, jump up, go to the windows, look out to make sure there are no cops there, then I sit back down for awhile. After another hit, it's the same thing all over again. I feel like a jack-in-the-box, only it's a little crazy too. I know they're not really out there, but I gotta make sure anyway.

Therapist: And that happens most of the time now?

Francine: Yeah, but I never think about that when I'm going to get the blow; I'm only thinking about getting high.

Therapist: What you're describing isn't very unusual. In fact, a lot of people get paranoid behind cocaine and think they're going nuts, when it's really a side effect of the coke. How did it used to be?

Francine: Well, at first it was great. I don't know. I just felt terrific. And I'd have these great conversations with my boyfriend. I liked it a lot. Then later I noticed what you mentioned before about that irritableness, and when I took all those pills I was depressed, real depressed, and that was only about an hour or so after I based.

Therapist: Okay, you've got it. Let me tell you a little about something called "cocaine psychosis." Ever heard of it?

Francine: No, [laughing] but it sounds bad. What is it?

Therapist: It can be bad, but luckily it isn't permanent. So even in its worst form, if the person stops using cocaine, they'll usually be back to normal within a couple of days. And it doesn't sound like you've had it real bad. It sounds like you've only experienced stage one and stage two.

Stage one is characterized by feelings of irritability, nervousness, depression, and a general letdown after doing cocaine. Most people who do cocaine more than a few times will experience stage one. In fact, that's where people start getting in trouble with other drugs. They'll drink or use Valiums, or even heroin to cut the edge off of a coke crash when stage one gets bad. And then they don't realize they're getting in trouble with a second drug. Sound familiar?

Francine: I guess I have been drinking more regularly. And I did have those Valiums . . .

Therapist: Did have?

Francine: The ones I took when I tried to kill myself.

Therapist: When was that?

Francine: About two weeks ago.

Therapist: That's pretty recent. How are you feeling about life now?

Francine: Still scared, but a little better.

Therapist: Good. Let's talk about this cocaine psychosis busi-
              ness, and then we'll get back to your depression,
              okay?

Francine: Okay.

Therapist: All right. So, I just told you about stage one. Now,
              stage two is characterized by paranoia. Just like what
              you were saying; where the person feels paranoid and
              knows there is no basis in reality for their paranoia,
              but they are still scared. That's what was happening
              when you were running to the windows. Also, in
              stage two the cocaine crash is worse. You are more
              irritable, more depressed, more on edge. So you see,
              when you took those pills two weeks ago, it wasn't
              really you taking them. It was you under the direct
              influence of a very powerful drug acting in a way
              you wouldn't, if you didn't have the drug working
              on you. You are probably okay, and I can assure you
              after talking with you for the last forty-five minutes
              that you're not crazy. The drug is crazy, but you're
              not.

Francine: Are you sure?

Therapist: Yup. When I worked at a clinic I used to do the
              psych evaluations, so I have a lot of experience in
              this. You're not crazy. You do have a drug problem.
              And if you want to feel "normal" again, whatever
              that means, you'll have to stop using. I'll help with
              that, and then we can work together on other prob-
              lems in your life—what all bothers you and gets you
              depressed, because we all get depressed at times.
              You'll be surprised, when you're drug free, how
              much easier it is to cope with things than when
              you're using and putting all those artificial highs and
              lows in your life. That's schizy and crazy-making.

Life itself is difficult enough without those extra bumps.

Francine: You're right on that one.

Therapist: Okay now, stage three. In stage three you lose track of the paranoia, and now you're sure that what you're paranoid about is real and is in fact happening. You get out of touch with reality. People have gone into uncontrollable rages, destroying things, tearing apart their apartment, beating someone up, screaming and hollering, and even committing suicide. Some of this actually may have been happening to you when you took those pills. You can get real dangerous to yourself or others during this stage. It's scary, but not permanent. I've seen people right after they've beat up their old ladies or pulled apart pieces of machinery with their bare hands. It can get ugly.

Francine: Yuck, I guess I've been lucky.

Therapist: Any questions?

Francine: No.

Therapist: Okay, I'll see you next week at the same time. And try each morning to think about what I said about the disease you have, and that the only recovery is abstinence. Then try to get through that whole day, just that day, without using. And do that each day. Just one day at a time. Here are lists of AA, CA, and NA meetings around the city. Try to go to at least three this week.

Francine: I don't like groups.

Therapist: That's okay. Try it anyway, it's an important part of your recovery program. It'll help you stay clean. You don't have to say anything, just go and listen.

Francine: Well . . . I'll try.

Therapist: That's all I can ask. We'll talk more about the meetings next week, but time's running out now. Okay, good luck, and remember it's not your fault. Have a good week and I'll see you next week. Oh, one more thing; if the urge gets real bad, give me a call, okay?

Francine: Thanks.

Therapist: Sure, see you soon.

Francine: All right.

Francine was a very cooperative client. She realized her life was out of control and that she was going to have to do something different. There was no denial present in her, only eagerness to find a different way of coping. Initial sessions like these can be very gratifying to both the therapist and the client. The therapist leaves feeling she has made an impact on the client. The client is ready to abstain from cocaine, although understandably anxious, now that she knows she has a disease that explains all the "craziness" that had been scaring her so much. The onus has been lifted.

Unfortunately, even after such an idyllic first session, the person may not be able to stay clean. So it is important to warn clients before they leave that if they use, they ought to mark down when it was, how much they used, and what the circumstances surrounding their usage were and then go on, rather than dwelling on it. I warn them that recovery from their disease takes a while. I tell people to be a little nicer to themselves if they do slip; they shouldn't beat themselves black and blue if they use again.

The first session is like launching a boat. You can fully equip it, but until the crew is trained they'll have a rocky trip. When these clients return and I find out when, how, and what they used, then I am beginning to get baseline data on what skills they may have for abstinence. I don't expect too much. I can try to figure out why they slipped in terms of trigger events or trigger moods; but addicts slip because they are addicts, people whose drug usage is out of control. That's why they're coming to therapy. So we don't dwell on the slips or possible explanations or justifications for them; instead, we talk more about recovery and what that is going to mean.

10. The Next Step Toward Recovery

When a therapist is sitting in her office, waiting for a cocaine abuser or addict to arrive for the second session, a number of possible scenarios may go through her mind: (1) he (or she) won't return, he's decided to continue using; (2) he'll come in and tell you he's been clean all week and feels great; (3) he'll come in and say he's been clean all week and it's been a real struggle to stay clean; (4) he'll have used at least once during the week and he's embarrassed about it; or (5) he'll come in and say the cocaine problem is fine, he hasn't touched it, and only had one beer with his pizza the other night. He will report that all is well. One of these five scenes is probably about to be played out.

"I'M NOT COMING BACK"

If clients do not show up, the therapist can call and find out why. Often the person does not answer the phone, so the therapist is stuck. When that happens I usually sit down, go over our first session in as much detail as I can recall, and ask myself what the client said and how I responded, looking for clues to explain this absence. I need to make sure, or in this way reassure myself, that I did my job; it's the client that is breaking our agreement.

It is amazing how often I have heard, (when I do reach the person), "Oh, geez, was that today? I could have sworn it was tomorrow, why I've got it in my book as tomorrow. Hey, I'm sorry, can we reschedule?" About 70 percent of these clients also miss this new appointment and never pay me for either one (despite my policy that people must pay for sessions that are not canceled with at least twenty-four-hours notice). These people are ready in their more lucid moments and know intellectually that they need help, but they are just too scared and not yet ready or willing to make a commitment to treatment (which will mean giving up all drugs).

I agree to see them when they are ready, and point to the futility of setting up a third appointment when their behavior has spoken very powerfully and is saying, "I'm not ready." I chalk these up to disappointments that are expected in this business, and I hope they will call again when they are ready and willing. To the therapist, this situation represents lost money, and a lost hour (or a free hour or two). It also may mean taking some time to feel badly that this person is going to have to hurt more before he allows himself to hurt less. By accepting that reality, the therapist can get off "the responsibility hook."

"I'VE BEEN CLEAN ALL WEEK AND I FEEL GREAT"

Sometimes clients will come in and tell me they've been clean all week and feel great; in this case I get to congratulate them, ask if they've noticed any changes this week, ask how they feel and how the world looks to them, and carefully plan how to keep them going. I always feel a need to remind people that it's great they've been clean for a week, but they can't get too cocky about that, because there are no reassurances that an initial clean week guarantees a clean life. They have simply taken their first step and need to continue down that path.

Therapist: So, how was it for you?

Frank: Real good. Actually, a little strange, too.

Therapist: Tell me about both those things—the good part and the strange part.

Frank: Well, let's see, the good part, it was OK. I actually was surprised how easy it was. I just stayed home and did what I had to do. I cleaned my apartment and ate well like you suggested. I cooked and I even went for a bike ride in Golden Gate Park. And I felt good that I was being good.

The strange part was that I thought I had to avoid my friends and it was strange when I ran into them on the street; I had to get away before they could offer me a **toot**. I wasn't sure if they would, but I was scared they might. I figured I was too new at this to know how to turn it down.

Therapist: So you needed to avoid friends to stay clean?

Frank: I thought I had to.

Therapist: Did you go to any meetings?

Frank: Well, I almost did. Really, I thought about it a lot, but I figured I was doing so well that I didn't have to go.

Therapist: But it sounds like you were doing well partially because you cut yourself off from people. That's certainly OK to do for a while. It sounds like you used the extra time to get your life a little more in order. I'm glad to hear you gave your body that extra nutritional attention; it probably needed that. And the exercise too. Those are two important components of your recovery.

Another component is getting some support through all this. Coming to see me once or twice a week just isn't enough. You're going to need more, especially if you're afraid your friends won't be able to be supportive—and that's not their fault. If they're as hooked into this drug as you've been, they aren't capable of helping you, they can't even help themselves; at least you got yourself in here.

Frank: I guess I see your point, but I can't do everything at once, I'm not perfect.

Therapist: Hey, you're right, and you know what? Neither am I. I didn't mean to imply that you had to be perfect. I'm just suggesting that even though it sounds like a lot of things to be doing all at once—eating well, exercising, coming here, going to meetings—all of that will maximize your chances of staying clean.

You have to put as much time and energy into staying clean as you used to put into getting high. We can't have you getting bored or listless right now, because your cure for that is still on automatic—cocaine—so we need to keep you busy for a while staying clean. Do you remember last week when I explained to you that a full recovery program included individual work, group work, and a family or couple's component if you had a partner or significant other? That's still all I'm asking you to do.

Frank Well, I was real proud of myself this week.

Therapist: And you had good reason to be. You did fine. Now let's talk about your upcoming week and let's see if we can make sure you do at least as well. I'm pushing these meetings for another reason besides just the people support—I honestly believe that the twelve-step program they offer will be tremendously helpful to you. It's something that's worked for millions of people. And I think it's worth checking out seriously.

Frank: OK. I see your point now. I guess I'm ready to try something else. You know, all this is so new for me . . . And I'm going on blind faith here. You're telling me what to do and I've got to believe you, but that's not so easy. I'm not used to just doing what someone else says.

Therapist: I understand that, and I'm glad to know how you feel. Hopefully, I won't be directing you for long. But for now, it's important that we plan together and that I tell you how to fill in the gaps. We want to try to let you take a rest. In a sense, your decisions are temporarily impaired by addictive thinking, and until we get your thinking and your actions back on the right track you're going to have to surrender the driver's seat. Don't worry, I have no intentions of making you permanently dependent. The last thing I want to do is think of what you should do with the rest of your life. I just want to get you in shape so you can handle your life when you're ready and have the resources to let go of what you can't handle.

You'll understand some more of what I'm saying in a few weeks, when your toxicity lowers and the drugs are no longer affecting your system; the meetings will also help. Until then, as you say, blind faith will guide you if you allow it.

Frank: I don't see that I have any choice really. My thinking—as you say, my addictive thinking—got me here. I can only hope yours is better.

Therapist: You've got the picture now. So are you going to add a few meetings to your recovery program this week?

Frank: OK.

Therapist: Good, I think you'll enjoy them.

Frank gave me a lot of information. Part of what I have learned is that he's going to need a lot of strokes for his accomplishments. He is also on the defensive much of the time; but if I don't react directly to that and validate where the defensiveness is coming from, I can get past it. In a sense, he is shaping how I need to act and react to him to make our treatment compatible with his personal style. More of that mutual feeling-out will be occurring for weeks.

His behavior and words show that he is anxious and scared about his recovery. These reactions are valid and need to be treated as valid and understandable. He needs to know that I'll respect and listen to his feelings and needs, that I'll take them into account, *and* that I'll stand up for what I believe to be therapeutically beneficial (including incorporating his needs into a more healthy recovery). He needs to know that I'm not a pushover, that my responsiveness and the program we outline is originated in clearheaded (chemical-free) thoughts and beliefs. He needs to trust that plan and follow it with some of that blind faith we talked about in the session.

"I'VE BEEN CLEAN ALL WEEK AND IT'S BEEN A REAL STRUGGLE"

Some clients will return and tell me they've been clean all week and it's been very difficult to remain clean. They have experienced "white knuckle sobriety," which is no fun at all. With white knuckle sobriety, a person, by sheer strength and continual battle, does not succumb to any drugs, but battles all the way. This active fight is very different from giving up drugs and being able to get through hours, days or even weeks at a time, not thinking about doing drugs. Let's look at what made it so hard for the client, and what he can do to make it easier and more pleasurable.

Charlie: Boy, you would have been proud of me. I did real good this week, but it was hard. Shit, I felt like I was fighting this continual battle. I never knew how pervasive drugs could be. They kept flooding in. It doesn't stay this bad, does it?

Therapist: Usually not, but those pervasive thoughts you're talking about are probably what we call "drug hunger," and they can persist for a long time.

Charlie: Oh, no. How long?

Therapist: Do you remember me telling you last week that you might experience drug hunger?

Charlie: Not really, but now that you mention it the term sounds familiar, so you probably did.

Therapist: Drug hunger is when thoughts, images, smells, or feelings associated with using invade your being and you find yourself wanting or craving the drug, involuntarily.

Charlie: That's it. I had it bad last week.

Therapist: That's a common reaction. It's your first attempt at staying clean. But it sounds like you're trying the "willful" method.

Charlie: Willful?

Therapist: You're trying to control yourself, to fight off the drugs at all odds by will power alone.

Charlie: Well, that's what I've got to do, isn't it?

Therapist: That's one way of going about it, but what you are trying is almost impossible to accomplish. Did you see *Star Wars* and its sequels?

Charlie: Three to five times each.

Therapist: Okay—remember how many years of training Luke Skywalker had to have before he could face Darth Vader? Well, you're trying to face Darth Vader with no training, with no support, and you expect to win? You've got to be crazy to put that expectation on yourself. Your only hope in that situation is to give up the fight and hope some higher power will come along and take care of you. You certainly do not have the power alone, you've proved that over time already.

Charlie: Are you saying, for me, drugs are my Darth Vader, and they are so obviously stronger than I that I shouldn't even attempt to fight?

Therapist: You've got it. Now I am not saying to go back to drugs—I'm not saying that at all. You have to admit that it's unmanageable, that your life and your drug use are out of control, and let it go.

Charlie: But don't I die then, don't I get overwhelmed by my opponent's force?

Therapist: No, not if you get a **higher power** to help you.

Charlie: What do you mean about a higher power? That sounds kind of weird.

Therapist: I mean some force greater than you, something you can believe in that knows more, is stronger than you.

Charlie: Look, I don't really like what you're saying. I don't believe in God and I've just got to be strong enough to fight what you call my "disease of addiction" on my own.

Therapist: Why?

Charlie: 'Cause I've always fought my own battles.

Therapist: Well, maybe it's time to stop . . .

Charlie: Huh?

Therapist: You came in here, didn't you? You're asking for my help, aren't you?

Charlie: That's different.

Therapist: Why?

Charlie: It just is.

Therapist: How is it different?

Charlie: I was just too tired, frustrated, and scared, and I guess I realized I was fighting a losing battle.

Therapist: Okay, so you admitted your own personal powers weren't enough.

Charlie: Yeah, I admitted it, but it's hard to stick to that realization.

Therapist: I understand that. It is hard sometimes, real hard for us to ask for help. Let's go back to what you said about not liking what I was saying because you don't believe in God. I'm not asking you to believe in God, and I'm not asking you to believe in some California hug-a-tree spiritualism; but something got you here . . . Something got you to realize you were fighting a losing battle, something got you, Mr. Indepentfighter, to ask for help. And maybe, just maybe, that something is your higher power.

Charlie: Oh, is that what you mean?

Therapist: Kind of.

Charlie: But that was easy; it just happened, I threw up my hands and somehow I heard about you, called you, and here I am.

Therapist: Yup, that's true, but what was that "something" that "just happened"?

Charlie: [Laughing] Okay, you got me. So you're suggesting I throw up my hands a little more often and admit defeat, that I can't control it, and see what happens.

Therapist: You've got it. I also suggest you come in here, eat well, exercise, go to meetings, give yourself congratulations for every day that you don't use, reward yourself in some way, be nice to yourself, and start to write about your progress.

Charlie: Write? I never kept a diary.

Therapist: Does that mean that because you never have, you can't now?

Charlie: No, not really, but I guess that is what I meant. Why do you want me to do that?

Therapist: It's helpful to have a personal running account of your progress, of how you feel, of how proud you are, of what's going differently in your life, how things are. It's nice to look back and see your progress in getting to know yourself and it'll help you during rough times ahead.

Charlie: Do you really think so?

Therapist: Yes, or I wouldn't be suggesting it. I know it's something else new, but with your history we need all the help we can get. And I know this has helped a lot of people. Just use it when you want to. You don't have to write in it every night, just when the urge hits you or when you're ruminating about something and need some clarity, writing will often help. After a while it'll become more familiar and you'll know when to do it.

Charlie: Well, maybe I'll try it.

Therapist: Is that all?

Charlie: What do you mean?

Therapist: Trying isn't enough, as my co-therapist, Tim Mc-Carthy, showed me the other day—try to stand up. [Client stands] You didn't try.

Charlie: What do you mean? I did so.

Therapist: No, you stood up.

Charlie: Well, I tried to. . . .

Therapist: Right, but the trying part was the effort alone, when you stood you weren't trying to stand, you were actually standing—do you see what I mean? It's the difference between trying and doing. One leads to a direct action, and the other may short-circuit a direct action.

Charlie: [Snickering] That's pretty good. I never thought of it like that.

Therapist: Neither had I; I really liked it too. Now let's go back to your original statement today.

Charlie: I don't remember what it was.

Therapist: You said that I would be really proud of you for staying clean this week.

Charlie: Well, aren't you?

Therapist: I'm glad for you, glad that you were able to experience a drug-free week, and I sure hope that continues and gets easier for you, but that's not the point. It's not for me to be proud of you, you're the important one here. Are you proud of yourself?

Charlie: Well, sure, but I was interested in your reactions.

Therapist: I understand, and that's part of the dependency needs we'll explore later on. They usually come hand in hand with addiction. We need to teach you how to give yourself your main goodies. So, at the end of the week, ask yourself how you feel about yourself, and have your reactions be important than anyone else's. To have you appreciating and having faith in yourself, in your feelings, in your judgments, so you don't have to look to another human being for validation; that will be quite an accomplishment for you.

Charlie: I never thought of it like that.

Therapist: That's okay. Give yourself a pat on the back for

seeing it now. Every time you learn something new, see if you can be pleased with yourself for letting that new knowledge in and not blocking it out. You've got to learn to like yourself, to be your best friend and confidant, to know you can count on yourself. For a long time now, you couldn't, because you were a "drug addict" and everyone knows you can't trust "those people." But now, get to know you, your core—it may be the first time you are clearheaded enough to look inside that far—certainly it's the first time since being an "adult." You may be surprised by what you find. It may even please you.

Charlie: You're probably right there.

Therapist: Well, test it out and tell me about it next week. We've got to stop now, we're runing out of time. . . . Good session. Thanks for being here.

Charlie: Being here?

Therapist: It was a heavy session and you hung in there well. See you next week. Have a good week.

Charlie: You too. And thanks a lot.

Therapist: You're welcome.

Charlie is less defensive than the previous client, Frank. He is open to new ideas, although his initial reactions are hesitant to negative. He seems to need a lot of reassuring, which usually suggests underlying insecurities. Addicts often start using drugs, especially cocaine, to hide or compensate for their own insecurities. They may have initially succeeded in hiding or masking their insecurities, but the reality of those insecurities comes rising to the surface as soon as the drugs are eliminated.

In addition to the original insecurities, new ones are added by addicts' guilt associated with their drug use. I have found that most people have internalized the public's reactions to "an addict" even if they have not openly admitted to being one. And because common knowledge says that "you can't trust an addict" (a piece of common knowledge that has a good deal of grounding in reality), addicts feel badly about themselves; they can't trust themselves and don't like themselves. I assume some of this dynamic is operating with Charlie.

In ensuing sessions I will have him identify and deal with his insecurities and his self-esteem by getting him to take note of his accomplishments and progress. One of my therapeutic goals for Charlie will be getting him to be more self-centered in a healthy fashion, so he isn't looking to others for approval and is therefore more independent. He needs to learn how to ask for help when he needs it (like coming to see me), and he needs to learn when to look inside for strength or to his own higher power. These will all be vital parts of his recovery and continued sobriety; when you like yourself, it's harder to be self-destructive.

This was a fast-paced session. Charlie kept feeding me information to work with, which I just had to keep track of and fire back at him. His responses were open and willing, even when he was hesitant. This kind of session is exciting, fun, and thought-provoking for me as the therapist, and for the client who leaves with his brain and guts challenged and fed. He even looks more alive; his cheeks have more color than when he walked in, and his eyes are sparkling and have more of a glow to them, may-be because he's letting himself hear some things he feels will help him. He sees hope for himself. Instilling hope is an impor-tant part of the beginning stages of recovery—hope that life can get better.

"I USED DURING THE WEEK, AND I'M EMBARRASSED"

Some clients will say that they've used during the week; they're generally embarrassed, upset, or defensive about it. I remind them that a slip during a first attempt at recovery is fairly com-mon, and I use it to reinforce the existance of the addictive disease; here they are, hell-bent on staying clean, and still they can't stay away from cocaine. I take more care in getting them to program their next week with healthy activities to minimize the chances of slipping again. Another important part of the session will be to look at what stopped them from doing the rest of the plan we had set up during the previous session.

Depending on the client's stance (defensive, embarrassed, or upset), I will respond accordingly. When clients are defensive, I may ask what's making them so cocky and say it's okay to be upset; they don't have to be right all the time; we drive ourselves crazy trying to be "right" all the time. If they are upset I may tell them they need the energy they're using on being upset to think and work more positively for sobriety, and to enjoy sobriety as they achieve it. When clients are embarrassed, I may tell them that it's understandable that they're embarrassed, but I'm not there to judge, only to help them in their quest and struggle for a chemical-free lifestyle.

Therapist: So, how was this past week for you?

Diane: Oh, pretty good.

Therapist: Pretty good? What does that mean?

Diane: It means pretty good. Why are you asking?

Therapist: I'm asking because I don't know what you mean by pretty good—it could mean almost anything. What do you mean?

Diane: Well, it means pretty good.

Therapist: We're not getting very far very quickly. You want to tell me what's bugging you?

Diane: This isn't working.

Therapist: This?

Diane: Therapy, goddamn it. I left here feeling real good last week. I was sure I was going to be okay, but it just didn't last. About three days later I got real depressed—I'm talking the pits—and then that night I went to my friend Gail's. She doesn't usually use much but she had some and before I could tell her what you said to do, about me not using anymore, she had offered me some and I had said "yes." I felt bad the next day, but then I just went out and copped some more so I'd feel better.

Therapist: And did you?

Diane: For a while. I think I'm going to give this up. I just can't afford to come here anymore.

Therapist: You mean you can't afford me and the coke.

Diane: Well . . .

Therapist: Come on, let's be honest here. Did you really think that after one visit you would be magically "cured" of a drug problem that has taken you six years to develop?

Diane: No, not the way you're putting it, no, I didn't think that, but it sure would be nice.

Therapist: I agree, it sure would be; but that's not possible. People often use after their first session.

Diane: Why?

Therapist: For lots of reasons. Perhaps the biggest is that they're addicts. You're an addict. You have a disease and your recovery is not an easy process. Sometimes it seems to me people also use to test themselves. "Can I actually use less? Can I control it? Is this really a disease that is out of control? Do I really have a problem?" And maybe they're also trying to prove that treatment won't work so they can feel justified in going out and continuing to use. And that's crazy, addictive thinking. Any of that sound familiar?

Diane: . . . Yeah, but I don't like to admit it.

Therapist: Why not?

Diane: Because I might have to keep coming, and it's hard.

Therapist: What's so hard about coming?

Diane: It makes my day so long, to come in here after work, and my boyfriend doesn't like it, that I'm coming here.

Therapist: Why not?

Diane: I'm not sure. . . . He does drugs too, and maybe he's afraid you'll tell me to leave him or something.

Therapist: Why do you say that?

Diane: What?

Therapist: That he's afraid I'll tell you to leave him?

Diane: I don't know.

Therapist: Well, that had to come from somewhere. Do you think you should leave him?

Diane: Sometimes . . . but I love him.

Therapist: Please make sure that you hear this loud and clear: I am not telling you what you should do with your boyfriend. Any of those doubts right now are coming from you. I wouldn't want that responsibility.

Diane: Okay, I understand.

Therapist: And about making your day too long—your days were a lot longer when you were using drugs every day and staying up most of the night.

Diane: That's true.

Therapist: So I can't accept the long day reason—that falls into the "bullshit excuse" category. You'll have to come up with something more legitimate to get my sympathy. Remember I told you you were going to have to spend the same amount of time getting clean as you used to getting high?

Diane: That's a lot of time.

Therapist: I know. Look, I never said this was going to be easy. I did say that I'd be there, every step you took, for guidance and support, but I never said it would be easy. Keep in mind what your life was like the week before last, when you were using every day. That wasn't easy either. You have your choice.

Diane: [Crying] Well, when you put it like that I see what you mean and what I have to do, only why can't I see things like that when you're not around?

Therapist: Why? Because you still have an active disease that affects your thinking . . . and you may not even be aware of some of your options because you've coped by using drugs for so long. That's why it's important for you to continue to come for treatment—so you can learn to think about different options and different ways of responding besides a quick drug-induced escape or high.

Diane: [Sniffling] I guess I agree, but what about my boyfriend?

Therapist: What about him?

Diane: He uses too.

Therapist: How much?

Diane: Not as much as me, he has it under control.

Therapist: Are you sure?

Diane: Yeah, but I guess I should watch it now that I'm not going to be using.

Therapist: That sounds like a good idea. . . . Do you think he could or would stop with you as support for what you're doing? Maybe for at least the first month?

Diane: I don't know. I could ask. He doesn't like therapy so much or me coming in here.

Therapist: You mentioned that earlier. Maybe we should talk about that a little. You seem concerned about it. But we also need to leave enough time to see how you're going to get through this next week and maximize your chances of staying clean so you can feel better.

Diane: Okay, that sounds like a good plan. Well, he thinks you're going to change me all around. His sister went to a therapist and then she got all uppity and he doesn't want me to get all uppity. Also, I think he's afraid I'll leave him.

Therapist: You know, I mentioned last week that a good way of doing outpatient recovery, which is what we are doing, is to bring in family members and friends. You refused to tell your family and I didn't realize you were so involved with your boyfriend—it would be a good idea if we got him in here, so he could see what we are doing, and who I am, and then he might not feel so left out.

Diane: He'd never come. He doesn't like therapy.

Therapist: He doesn't have to like it to try it. You could ask him as a favor to you, because you think we need his help and involvement. Otherwise, if we are battling him and your addiction the whole way, we're in for some trouble.

Diane: Well, I'll talk to him. It is pretty embarrassing, this whole thing. He fell in love with a healthy girl and now he has to know I have this disease that you say will never go away.

Therapist: Oh, so you haven't even told him yet?

Diane: No, did you think I did?

Therapist: From the way you were talking, yes. He does know you are coming to therapy?

Diane: Oh yeah, I told him that I was having some problems. I think he knows it's the cocaine.

Therapist: But you haven't told him directly?

Diane: No.

Therapist: What's stopping you?

Diane: I don't know.

Therapist: You don't know? I bet you could think about it and come up with something. Like maybe when you were saying that he's afraid you'd leave him, maybe you're really afraid he'd leave you.

Diane: I don't want to talk about it.

Therapist: I understand that this is hard for you, but it's real important that we get through this. If you have been using a lot with your boyfriend—or even if he is around you a lot—he is, whether you like it or want it, an important part of your recovery.

Diane: Don't you see? I'm embarrassed to tell him, just like I was embarrassed to tell you I slipped.

Therapist: I do see that. But one day you'll understand there is nothing for you to be embarrassed about. You have a problem and its cause is beyond your control; it has nothing to do with you, the essence or the core of you, it's a disease. It has affected your behavior, that's true. But once you are living a drug-free life that annoying and embarrassing behavior will no longer be in the picture. You need that energy that you're using on being embarrassed, upset, and angry to help you in your recovery program. Every day that energy could be transferred to begin the day by saying, "Today I won't use any drugs, today I'm going to be drug free." That energy can be used for you in more healthy and helpful ways.

Now let's go on and look at your week. One of your tasks is going to be to tell your boyfriend about what's really happening in your life. At least then you'll know where you stand and you won't have to be worrying. If you want, you can bring him in here and I'll help you tell him so I can explain some of this stuff about the disease that you may not be familiar with or feel comfortable with. But one of your first steps to recovery is admitting that you are an addict and openly admitting it to important people who you can trust, so you can get their support. You need to take some risks and take that first step.

Also, you have to go to three meetings this week.

Diane: Do I have to?

Therapist: Do you really want to clean up?

Diane: Yes, but . . .

Therapist: "Yes buts" don't work here. If it's "yes," then you'll go to meetings. Not going didn't seem to work too well last week.

Diane: But I thought coming here . . .

Therapist: I told you last week coming here once or even twice a week wasn't enough. Do you remember what I said about a full recovery program and maximizing your chances for a successful recovery?

Diane: You said I had to come here, go to meetings, tell my dealers not to sell me any, tell my friends I have a problem and can't do it anymore, and get my family to help too.

Therapist: Good, so you were listening. Now what's stopping you from doing all that?

Diane: I'm scared.

Therapist: You know, it's natural to be scared. We're talking about major changes in the use of your time, we're talking about changing the quality of your life. See if you can change some of that fear into being excited and anticipating a better life. That'll help you a lot.

Diane: Do you think so?

Therapist: Fear alone never killed anyone—you've got to face and walk through those fears. I know it's hard and I also know it's possible. Fear doesn't kill, but cocaine and alcohol do kill, and that's a fact. Now let's go back to your week. What are you going to do tomorrow?

Diane: Work.

Therapist: And then?

Diane: Maybe I'll go talk to Gail?

Therapist: Are you asking me or telling me?

Diane: [Nervous laugh] I'm telling you, I'll go.

Therapist: And after that?

Diane: I think I'll write in a journal, like you suggested.

Therapist: Good. And the next day?

Diane: Work, and maybe I'll go to a meeting.

Therapist: [With a smile] What's with all these maybe's?

Diane: Oh, you know . . .

Therapist: I do?

Diane: I guess I'm still trying to weasel out a bit.

Therapist: You'd better decide if you're making a commitment to this or not. It doesn't seem like your old self-esteem can use a lot more bruises. It seems battered and frail enough right now.

Diane: . . . When you said that, I felt like crying, like someone else knows how I feel. . . . I always play the big, strong role. You had mentioned maybe seeing me twice a week. Could we try that?

Therapist: I would be glad to. I think especially at the beginning you could use that support. What about Mondays and Thursdays? That gives a good spread, and we'll get you at the beginning of the week and toward the weekend.

Diane: Could I see you on Monday and Friday?

Therapist: Sorry, I don't see people on Fridays. Thursday is the latest day in the week we can meet.

Diane: Okay.

Therapist: If you haven't told your boyfriend by Thursday, let's role-play it, exchanging places. You'll be him or you, and I'll play both roles too. That way you can dress-rehearse it, see different ways of approaching him, and get more comfortable with the whole idea.

Diane: That sounds like a good idea.

Therapist: Okay, so in between now and Thursday you are going to how many meetings?

Diane: One.

Therapist: That means that between Thursday and Monday you'll need to go to two meetings.

Diane: All right, I'll go to two meetings.

Therapist: Okay. And if you get the urge to use you can call me, CA, NA, AA, or the National Council on Alcoholism. They're all listed in the phone book. The resources are there, all you have to do is use them.

Diane: I feel better, thanks.

Therapist: You're very welcome. Also, thank yourself. You did a lot of hard work today. Remember, these good feelings are like waves; they'll come and go and so will the bad ones. Try to ride them through, and give a call if you need help.

Diane: Thanks, see you Thursday.

Therapist: Right.

This session shows how vulnerable clients think they are when they are beginning treatment. At the beginning of the hour Diane had been ready to leave just because her first week had been hard and she'd slipped. After some reassurances and exploring what her options are if she continues to use (being miserable from the negative effects of the cocaine—the negative emotional, financial, and physical effects that she knows so well), she dropped her embarrassment and her defensiveness. This is not to say they are gone forever and her treatment will go smoothly from here. On the contrary, treatment is usually a rocky process, especially on an outpatient basis where you do not have the luxury of intense peer group and professional group support for remaining clean, and the addict's environment is not clean. That's why I try to get clients to get as much support from their environment as possible. They have a hard, but not impossible job ahead of them.

When clients start talking about not coming back, it is important for the therapist to keep her own ego from getting involved. The therapist needs to listen to the fears and justifications for not coming back, validate those, and then offer the alternative to not continuing—which, in effect, is the therapist's professional perspective. And if the person is really not ready to make a commitment to being completely drug free, then it is probably better for him or her to wait until they are ready; otherwise, both client and therapist are working in an impossible set of circumstances, and ultimately both will fail and both will feel badly. The therapist can get over this type of situation fairly easily—after all, she's not responsible for the client's outcome. But it's a lot harder on the client. The last thing in the world addicts need is another failure. They've already had far too many of those; it would just drop their self-esteem another notch or two and make it harder for them to try again at a later date. If, on the other hand, the therapist terminates treatment, making it clear that she is perfectly willing to resume whenever the client is willing, then therapy ends on a better note and makes it easier for the client to return.

"MY COCAINE PROBLEM IS FINE, I HAVEN'T TOUCHED IT—AND I ONLY HAD ONE BEER WITH MY PIZZA"

This is one of my favorites. It used to irk me no end, because I wondered why what I had said during the first session seemed to have so little effect once the person left my office. When I'd hear a client say those words, I would wonder if I had forgotten to talk about the disease model; then I'd quickly realize that was not a possibility, and would chalk it up to the "great eraser." This elusive force seems to invade people's minds, erasing away valuable tidbits of information and sometimes even substituting new pieces of information, like, "I'm different, I'm part of that 2 percent that can drink and not do cocaine after being a cocaine addict."

That great eraser used to frustrate me a lot. Now I simply accept its existence and begin where the client is—in denial—and go from there; only now I don't resent going over old territory; it simply becomes part of this client's recovery process.

Sometimes I ask clients to tell me what they remember that I said about the disease of addiction. Often they remember it all, especially the 2 percent exception, and they are hell-bent on proving to me and themselves that they are part of that lucky 2 percent. Others don't remember a whole lot at all (these are usually people who had often been under the influence when I'd first seen them); others may have been clean at the time, but their great eraser had been particularly effective.

At this point I reiterate my stance: I can only help them if they will agree to be drug free, and that includes being alcohol free. If they are not, we are fighting a losing battle, and I explain that I don't want to be part of that. I let them know, in no uncertain terms, that recovery is difficult enough without complicating it further with drugs. At this point, if they are still drinking or using other drugs, I will work with them for four to six weeks. At that time they have to make a commitment to live drug free, or we need to terminate treatment.

Therapist: So, how was your week?

Greg: Great.

Therapist: Good, that's nice to hear. . . . What made it great?

Greg: [Greg responds excitedly, with a big smile and glistening eyes] Well, it was my first week in six months without cocaine, and I really enjoyed it. It was easier than I thought and I enjoyed feeling more emotionally stable—more in control.

Therapist: That sounds like a terrific change. You certainly look real excited about that.

Greg: I am.

Therapist: What about other drugs?

Greg: Other drugs?

Therapist: Like alcohol and marijuana?

Greg: Oh, well, no problem, I told you that last week.

Therapist: Oh, then you didn't use any of those drugs?

Greg: Well . . . I told you last week, I don't have a problem with alcohol, I'm not an alcoholic. I didn't have any problems with it this week, I just had a beer with my pizza.

Therapist: Then you can't say you've been clean this week.

Greg: Oh, come on, one beer, that's no big deal.

Therapist: One beer may be no big deal for most people, but it is a big deal for you.

Greg: You're the only one making it into a big deal.

Therapist: That's true, but that doesn't make me wrong. I'm making it into a big deal because it is a big deal. When you are addicted, any drug—and alcohol must be included as a drug—can serve as a trigger for cocaine use.

Greg: But I didn't use cocaine this week.

Therapist: I understand that, but that is not to say you won't use it again. In fact, I can just about guarantee that if you continue to drink you will use cocaine again.

Greg: Oh, come on, I'm not talking about getting drunk, only one or two beers with my pizza or if I go to a club.

Therapist: That's one or two beers too many. You are honestly toying with a lot more trouble than you realize.

Greg: Huh?

Therapist:	We talked about the disease model last week. Let me review that with you again. [I go over it again.]

Greg: I just don't like it.

Therapist: That's obvious.

Greg: What do you mean?

Therapist: You're having a hard time accepting this reality of not being able to drink anymore. And what I call the "great eraser" seems to have invaded your brain and wiped the slate clean, because we talked about the disease model last week. It's okay, it happens pretty often; I see it more as a measure of your denial working.

Greg: But I'm not denying that I have a cocaine problem.

Therapist: In a way you are, because you are not accepting the more far-reaching effects of having a cocaine problem.

Greg: I lost you again.

Therapist: [Smiling] I know, that's your old denial blocking me out again. When you're an addict you are addicted to all drugs, in a sense: All drugs can trigger a relapse to your drug of choice. That may not happen the first couple of times you have your "one beer," but it'll happen somewhere down the road.

Greg: I don't believe it.

Therapist: You don't believe it, or you don't want to believe it?

Greg: Does it matter?

Therapist: Yes, it does in terms of how far you can get in this recovery program. If you don't believe it and you are going to maintain that stance, then I can't help you. If, on the other hand, you just don't want to believe it, then I may be able to help you work through that and begin your recovery program.

Greg: But I did begin this week.

Therapist: No, sorry, you think you began a recovery program, but you did not begin a legitimate recovery program that has some good chances of working. To do that you have to be committed to what I outlined to you last week.

Greg: But I went to two CA meetings and I really liked them.

Therapist: Good, but that still does not address the issue of being drug free. The meetings won't help in the long run if you're still drinking. . . . If you liked the meetings, why not go back and talk up and ask people what they've found about the necessity of a drug-free lifestyle in their recovery. Ask them—don't just take my word for it.

Greg: I don't want to.

Therapist: Why not?

Greg: Because I know what they'll say.

Therapist: What'll they say?

Greg: They'll agree with you.

Therapist: So?

Greg: I don't want to have to stop drinking. That's not my problem. It seems like I should be able to still do that. I need some fun and relaxation in my life.

Therapist: I understand this is very hard for you, and you're probably feeling deprived already from eliminating the cocaine.

Greg: That's right!

Therapist: Hold on, let me finish, because you just put out a lot of stuff in your last statement and I want to address each issue. It all flowed out so quickly that it's probably all important stuff.

Drinking may not have been your problem, but addiction is your problem. And because of that, drinking has now become an indirect-direct problem. Indirect in that it will trigger further cocaine use, and direct in that you must stop drinking to prevent more cocaine problems. I know that it "seems" like you should be able to still use it, I agree that it seems that way. But things are not always as they seem, and this is one of those instances.

People often get angry and take the "why me?" stance, which is valid. "Why do I have to stop drinking when that wasn't ever a problem?" Well, nobody ever said life was going to be fair, and in one sense, you're one of the lucky ones who gets to learn to live a drug-free life. And there are lots of benefits to that, if you'll let yourself experience it for a while and do what I suggest.

In terms of having fun and relaxing, amazingly enough, there are other ways than through drugs. If you'll bring in a cassette recorder and a sixty-minute tape I'll make you a relaxation tape you can use and we can brainstorm a lot of other things you can do to have fun and relax. It is possible.

Greg: Hmm, what you're saying makes sense, but I still don't want to stop drinking.

Therapist: You know you can not want to, but still not drink.

Greg: Somehow it wasn't as hard to say that I'll never do cocaine again as it is for me to say I'll never drink again.

Therapist: Then don't say never, just start each day by saying, "Today I won't have a drink."

Greg: I said that today. There's a birthday party at work today, and I already decided I wasn't going to drink at that just so I could see how it feels.

Therapist: That's a first step. . . . But there's something strange about all this for me . . .

Greg: What do you mean?

Therapist: Well, if alcohol has not been a problem for you, as you say, and you drink very little, I'm wondering why it is that something that is not important to you is so hard to give up? Isn't that contradictory?

Greg: [Nervous laugh] Yes, but like you said, I don't want to feel deprived.

Therapist: Hey, if you want to feel better about being deprived, think of the starving people in Namibia.

Greg: [Laughing] But at least they can drink if they want.

Therapist: [Smiling] But they can't eat or drink much, even if they want to. You are making a free choice to live a long and healthy and happier life; but they have no choice. And like my father always used to say when I was a little girl, "It's always good to want something."

Greg: Did your father really say that?

Therapist: Yes, all the time, and I hated it at the time. But as an adult I have appreciated learning that at an early age.

Greg: Hmmm, I guess that would have been helpful. I always feel deprived and upset when I want something and can't have it. But if I felt like it was okay to want something and not get it, I might not be as depressed.

Therapist: That's probably true. So what's it going to be with the alcohol?

Greg: Do I have to decide now?

Therapist: Now's as good a time as any. You have all the facts and you are fully aware of the alternatives.

Greg: I don't like being pushed.

Therapist: I gathered that already. You like to be in control. Guess what, you're not . . . why don't you let this one go too? I can guarantee it will make your life easier.

Greg: Well shit, what about if I just see what it's like for a while? I'm not saying that I think it's necessary, I just want to prove to you and the people at CA that it's not important.

Therapist: Seeing what it's like to be drug free for a month is okay with me. We'll talk about it as we go and see how you are finding it . . .

In this case I did not get a firm commitment, but I felt that I would within the month. Greg's last statement did not make a lot of sense, and seemed to indicate to me that he was unhappily going along with eliminating alcohol from his life. But as long as he did that, kept going to meetings, and came in for therapy, I was pretty sure he'd convince himself. I made sure that he continued attending CA meetings regularly and kept track of his progress and his feelings as the "experimental month" progressed.

Sometimes I have had to go through sessions like this repeatedly for a few weeks, and in some cases for a few months. At this point, however, I will not continue to treat a client who does not want to be drug free after six weeks of treatment. Months of arguing is not very effective; so when it looks like we're into a battle of wills or a battle for control, I give up and step out.

Therapist: Look, this is not working and it is not going to
work. You are convinced that you can drink and still
control your cocaine use, and I'm convinced that you
can't. You pay me to know more about this stuff
than you, but then you don't trust me or do what I
am suggesting. I can't help you, given those circumstances. It's impossible. I'd like to help you, but
you're not giving yourself or me a chance.

I tell you what. Let's meet for two more weeks
with the goal of terminating treatment until you are
ready to start. I know when you walked in here four
weeks ago you thought you were ready, but your
behavior and your denial over the last four weeks
indicates that you're not. You're probably going to
have to go out there and bottom out some more and
think about what we've said during our sessions and
get more willing—you'll be looking at blind faith
when you come back—and compared to where you've
described you've been [staying up all night guarding
the house from people you imagined were going to
break in], it's got to be an improvement.

I want you to know, loud and clear: I am not
refusing to work with you; you are refusing to work
with me. And I'll be available when you're ready and
willing to work. Right now it seems too scary and
hard to you, and your denial is overriding the survivor in you that wants to feel better. I hope you'll be
back.

In the next two weeks we can wrap things up for
now, and talk about your fears and denial and try to
put all this into some perspective. If at the end of the
two weeks you're ready to be drug free, then we'll
renegotiate and continue to work together; if not,
we'll stop seeing each other until you want to return.

Please know you will be welcome back at any
time. I just don't want to give you false hope right
now. You don't need another failure. You're not ready,

and that's okay; you probably will be after you've experienced more pain, but let's save ourselves the pain of an unsuccessful attempt when it's doomed to failure.

It has taken me a long time to come around to this drug-free stance so early in treatment. But I have just seen too many unpleasant consequences of a more flexible attitude. Every person who has used other drugs during therapy with me has slipped and started to use cocaine again, which has made them feel even more worthless and hopeless, and that just isn't necessary. I don't want to lose clients that way. When I work with people now, they must be treatment ready or be able to get ready fast. If they aren't ready after six weeks, they need to go back out there and do whatever they are going to do until they are ready.

In some ways this stance has made my job harder, because people do not like to hear that they have to give up all drugs, even those they feel they don't have problems with. But what I have seen over the last three years has convinced me that I have no other ethical choice. I might add that for a private practitioner depending solely on a private practice for income, this method is not a great financial boon; but as a drug specialist who has my clients' interests at heart (and I've learned that their interests require a drug-free life), I know that anything short of this is probably not going to be a very effective recovery program. Some treatment facilities will not even begin to work with anyone who is not drug free; I have not gotten there yet, although I may. As an outpatient therapist, I will work with a client who's not yet clean, but only for about six weeks (because I think even that may be pushing it). A short treatment-ready phase is sometimes justified; and as my last example shows, in some cases working with someone while they get treatment ready is justifiable, as long as you limit the time allowed and make the expectations very clear to the client from the start.

Therapist and client have now made it through two sessions. Will there be a third, or a fourth? What will they be like? Sometimes it is more of the same, with a lot of "poor me" and "why me?" questions at the beginning. Then feelings begin to surface. Addicts are not familiar with having feelings, especially uncomfortable ones; they are even unaccustomed to good feelings. In some ways they are like babes in the woods, not quite knowing how to react. Once they are hooked into recovery and fully participating in all components, then they begin to learn how to deal with the feelings as they come. That is the subject of the next chapter.

11. Maintaining Sobriety

By the middle stage of treatment the therapist and client have succeeded in getting past the initial questions of, "Am I going to be in recovery?" and "Am I going to give up drugs?" The client has decided yes on both counts, has stopped using drugs, has learned about the disease model, and has made recovery the number one commitment in his or her life. At this time much of the struggle is over. The client has learned—initially by blind faith and later by questioning and planning with me, the therapist—to trust me, that I know what I'm doing; sessions now are more cooperative than they had been at the beginning of treatment.

During the middle stage of treatment the focus of each session will not be on the client's drug abuse per se, but on dealing with the consequences of this drug abuse and on generating new ways of behaving that are healthier and make them feel better than their old drug-related ways. At this time issues that involve other people often come up. For married people, the spouse often begins to get tired of all the meetings (AA, CA, NA) the addict has to go to, and his or her initial understanding is beginning to wear thin. Issues that come up for single people include, "How do I date?" "When do I tell a person I don't drink?" "Do I have to make an issue of my addiction right off the bat, or what?" People are very anxious about how to resume their social lives in a way that will be compatible with their recovery. Another issue that often comes up is the problem of how to deal with parents, some of whom are alcoholics and addicts themselves. During the initial phase of recovery, almost all the person's energy is focused on staying clean. During the middle stage the person is ready to consider a few more people and wants to know how to do that well.

At this point clients may begin to reduce the number of meetings they are attending each week, and it's very important for both client and therapist to watch the consequences of that reduction. Sometimes it is okay to drop down to two or three meetings a week if there are no negative consequences in their behavior or feelings. At this time a support group that consists of other newly recovering people may be very helpful for learning new social skills and how to interact without drugs. A support group based on the disease model (which also deals with the twelve step programs) can be very effective in increasing people's ease in social interactions and learning new ways of communicating. As one person said, "I'm dreading going dancing, something I always used to love to do, but I haven't done it straight since I was about fifteen; I don't know how I'll do it without any drugs. I'll probably be real self-conscious and stiff at first." The people I work with have associated all their good times with being high, and now they have to learn how to have good times without drugs.

In this middle stage it's important to check out any upcoming events or anniversaries of events that might be "triggers" to drug use. A trigger is an emotionally laden experience that previously would have been a perfect excuse, justification, or reason for getting high or increasing a person's usage. Trigger events could be the death of a parent or friend, the anniversary of a wedding or a divorce, or the anniversary of a rape. A trigger can also be a new or upcoming event—such as seeing a parent that one hasn't seen for years, having a sibling get married when the addict is single and would also like to be getting married. These kinds of issues can trigger drug use because that is how the addict has been accustomed to coping with emotional events—going away through drugs. It is important to anticipate these events and to discuss alternative (non-drug) ways to handle them. A person who has a variety of options available will be a lot less likely to use drugs.

If clients use during the middle phase of treatment, we talk about it but don't dwell on it. The important thing is that they are honest about their slips, and then get right back into the recovery program. They can use a slip as a further example of how unmanageable their life is and how powerless they are over drugs. With that information they may have to go to more meetings, or perhaps increase therapy sessions. If they begin to slip on a somewhat regular basis, then it is important to reexamine their recovery program and see what's missing (keeping in mind that an ideal recovery program includes an individual, a group, and a family component). Rather than reinforcing slips by paying too much attention to them, we look at the lessons to be learned from them and dwell more on progress to date and how to build on that. I keep in mind that addiction is a chronic, progressive, and relapsable disease; slips are viewed in that context, and I try to get clients to accept them and move on with renewed commitment to their recovery.

Addicts who continue to go to meetings and work on their recovery program usually make new friends through AA, NA, or CA. These new friends all share the same commitment to sobriety; but people they meet during day-to-day life do not know about recovery, and addicts may not know how to deal with them. There is a professional and personal side to this problem. What do addicts say at a business luncheon where everyone is ordering a drink? Often the first time is uncomfortable, but they get more and more used to saying, "I'll have a Perrier," or, "No, thank you," when the wine carafe gets passed around. Newly recovering people are concerned and often wonder if they need to give explanations about their non-drinking behavior; that should be talked about in therapy. In dating situations or on special occasions where drugs or alcohol are likely to be offered, it is helpful if the addict has already dress-rehearsed how to refuse because then the person can be more comfortable when this occurs in real life.

The middle stage of treatment can be a very heartening experience. Individual treatment is an important component of a continuing recovery program; by the middle stage of recovery the family members should ideally be involved with their own recovery programs. During this stage I give a lot of support to clients for remaining clean. Periodically, we review the progress they have made; by praising themselves, they reinforce these changes. We also talk about how their lives have changed, and how they are incorporating the twelve-step program in day-to-day living. We talk about and rehearse ways of finding new friends and having drug-free fun, continuing to explore new options for their newly acquired drug-free lifestyle.

This middle phase begins at various times, depending upon how long it takes a person to begin an effective recovery program. Some are ready to tackle these issues after being clean eight weeks, while others may take six months or a year. I do not rush people; rather, I try to validate their own rate for "getting there," as long as getting "there" involves staying on the road to recovery and not using. I will know they are on their way to recovery when they show me that they are sincerely willing; when they are going to meetings, when they are asking questions, and when they are beginning to look more optimistically at their lives. This chapter will present examples of each component of the middle stage of treatment.

INDIVIDUAL TREATMENT

In this situation, the client—"Michael"—is just beginning to "come alive again," and he's excited about the changes in himself and about what he is noticing around him. He has been clean for a little over two months, after having struggled for about two months over the decision to give up all drugs entirely. Finally, when I had told him that I couldn't help him anymore unless he was willing to stop doing drugs completely and start going to AA, NA, or CA meetings regularly, he finally decided to try what I was suggesting. He had reached the end of his rope and mine.

At the time of this session I had been working with him for a little over four months. This man, a thirty-five-year-old computer whiz, was just beginning to get back on his feet after losing his house because he couldn't make the mortgage payments, and having his girlfriend walk out on him as the house was being repossessed. He had managed to hold onto his job, although he was on probation there, and was trying to solidify his single life.

Michael: This is getting to be great. I mean, I feel better and better everyday, and today—today is just incredible.

Therapist: Oh yeah? What's so good?

Michael: [Agitated, excited] Well, noticing the world around me . . . for the last few days I've been noticing all these things that have always been around me, but that I stopped seeing years ago. It's been quite exciting. It's like the world is emerging again.

Therapist: Tell me some more.

Michael: Well, basically, I didn't know I could feel so good. I honestly didn't. I can't believe that I fought you so hard for two months when all you were trying to get me to do was experience this. I never want to forget how great I feel right now, never! This is just something else. I just feel so alive. When I wake up in the morning, I want to get up. I mean I'm actually looking forward to starting a new day. My friends who I used to use with wouldn't believe me if they heard me right now; honestly, they would think I had flipped out for sure. But I love it.

I feel more high today driving around and noticing trees and nice houses than I did for the last few years of using. But I couldn't stop then even though I wanted to lots of times. And I almost didn't stop now. It seems real important for me to remember how I feel today. I don't want to lose this. I'm afraid of what'll happen if I lose it.

Therapist: What are you afraid of?

Michael: [Sounding hyper] I'm afraid I'll slip. I really am. I want to stay feeling this good forever.

Therapist: Well, I hate to tell you this, but then again I better: You're not going to feel this good, this high all the time; it's unrealistic. And you need to know that, because as much as I don't want to burst your bubble, I do want to remind you about reality—or when you drop it might be very painful and disappointing to you. I can, however, pretty much guarantee that when you stick with your program you will have more days and periods of feeling good than you ever had before.

Feelings come in waves; remember me telling you that earlier? The good waves come and go, the bad waves come and go, the exhilarating waves come and go, the whole gamut of feelings comes and goes. It's great that you're noticing these things and feeling good. You sound a little high, and my concern is with the hyper quality of what you're saying. It sounds a little like when you were loaded, and that concerns me.

Michael: I'm not loaded!

Therapist: I know that, but I'm just saying please be prepared for the drop or that roll out. It's okay to feel good and even great, as long as you know that to expect to or want to feel like this all the time is unrealistic. It's that desire that got you in trouble once before. Right now you seem to be riding on the "pink cloud" of recovery. You need to allow yourself to feel all emotions and to enjoy them, even sadness and fear and strength and excitement. They are all valid in their own rights. To only want to feel one emotion is dangerous. Besides, look at all you would be missing out on. Do you see my point?

Michael: Yeah, I do. I guess what you're saying is that when I want to feel good all the time, or great and kind of high like now, that's what you've referred to as my "crazy addictive thinking," right?

Therapist: That's certainly one aspect of addictive thinking.

Michael: Well, at least I heard you that time and didn't fight you. I see your point. I can feel awful and now I can feel great, but feeling good or okay or nice, those are pretty nonexistent inside me. I guess I need to work on those mid-range emotions some more.

Therapist: You will. We'll work on it and you need to have some patience with yourself. You'll get there. You've only been clean for two months. You're still a babe in the woods in some ways. You've been using since . . . ?

Michael: Since I was fifteen—that's twenty years. I guess I have a lot to learn.

Therapist: And a lot to re-learn. It won't all be from scratch. Some you'll recognize from pre-fifteen. Just have some patience. Remember the serenity prayer?

Michael: Yeah—"God grant me the serenity to accept the things I cannot change, courage to change the things I can, and wisdom to know the difference."

Therapist: So, can you say that when you begin to get frustrated with yourself? And when you want it all "NOW"?

Michael: I do say it sometimes, but I could try to remember and say it a little more often.

Therapist: I think you're doing real well, considering where you were a mere four months ago—to say nothing of where you were a mere two months ago. I wasn't sure you were going to get into recovery or if you were going to end treatment when I gave you that ultimatum. And you decided to begin recovery. Today you're proud of yourself, grateful to be able to feel this way, and a lot happier than you were two months ago; that's a lot. No wonder you were so excited today. Just remember reality and try not to get so high that you can't see the ground.

Michael: Got it . . .

Often, feeling emotions that have not been felt in a long time becomes an issue we deal with in therapy. The person has been too stoned and too miserable to feel excited, happy, or even good. As this client said, he hadn't noticed everyday sights in a long time. His main focus for many years had been drugs—buying them, using them, and recovering from them. We talked about his excited feelings as well as possibilities of other emotions. He was frustrated when he didn't know what he was feeling; since an emotional response was so new for him, sometimes he couldn't identify how he was responding. He had to learn about responses and feelings all over again.

GETTING FAMILY MEMBERS INVOLVED

Ideally, we involve the person's family in recovery right from the start; they then can learn about the addictive disease and how it has affected them. That provides them with the option of beginning their own recovery programs. But, as in life, recovery doesn't always occur in an ideal situation; so at every opportunity presented, the therapist tries to encourage the addict to bring in significant others.

One of my clients, "Jim," had been very reluctant to involve his wife in his recovery. He said, "We don't have any problems, she hasn't been aware of the extent of my drug use, and she's felt no pain from it. I told her what you said I should tell her; she knows I can't drink or do drugs anymore, and she usually supports that. I don't want to bring her in here and rock the boat." That had been his stance every time I brought up the possibility of including his wife. I knew they were having some communication problems, but he was not willing to open up "that can of worms." His response was, "I know we don't talk, and if it ever gets bad enough I guess we'll have to. But right now we both seem to be all right with the silence." I had to accept his desires.

One day Jim told me about an upsetting experience that occurred when he had been clean for about seven months. He and his wife had gone out to their favorite restaurant for their anniversary. Over the years they had become friends with the owners who, in honor of their anniversary, had sent a good bottle of champagne over to their table.

Jim: Before I could say anything the waiter had appeared with the bottle, opened it up, and was beginning to pour it into the glasses on the table. I didn't know what to do. I knew I shouldn't drink it, but I did not want to insult the owners. I also didn't want to tell them why I couldn't drink it. And to make matters worse, they weren't there, and I knew the waiter would report to them what our response was. I must have looked visibly upset because my wife leaned over and said, "Don't worry, I'll drink it."

It was a relief that she was so understanding at the time, but I felt pretty foolish. I knew intellectually that I was doing the right thing, but I felt foolish; to not even be able to drink a glass of champagne with my wife on our anniversary. . . .

The next morning, as soon as I got up, I knew I had to go to a meeting. I got up and started getting ready for a brunch meeting when my wife said, "What are you doing?" I told her I was going to go to a meeting and she said, "After last night you are going to go to a meeting? But you didn't drink any of the champagne. I wish you'd just stay home with me. It's our one day to be together. Come on back to bed."

Well, I didn't have the heart to insist that I needed a meeting after she had been so understanding the night before, and it was clear her understanding was running out. I already felt guilty because I couldn't join her in a toast to us, so I went back to bed. It was a pretty unrelaxed day. Finally, I called one of the people I know from Alcoholics Anonymous and talked to him for a while. Then I felt a little better. I know I can't expect my wife to understand completely, but I wish she had been more understanding . . .

Therapist: Do you wish you could have explained to her better why you felt a need to go to a meeting Sunday morning?

Jim: Sure.

Therapist: Well, there are two ways to handle that. One way is for us to practice ways you can talk to her. And the other—and, I might add, the more effective way—is to get her in here and we can work with her in person. You know, she has some feelings and needs too, and if she doesn't express those to you at home we can only pretend we know what they are. It makes it harder to decide what you could be saying to her so she understands more.

Jim: You've got a point; let me think about it.

Therapist: What do you have to think about?

Jim: If I want to take the risk.

Therapist: Keep in mind that all the other risks you've taken so far have worked out pretty well.

Jim: Hmm . . .

Therapist: I have a feeling, and correct me if I'm wrong, that part of what keeps you from bringing her in here is your reluctance to go public with your addiction. One of the options you had at the restaurant was to tell the waiter, "Thank you very much, but I don't drink." And you were very upset lest he know you couldn't drink. You also indicated when you were talking that you didn't want the owners to know, and you were concerned that if you refused the champagne you would insult them. If they'd known why you had refused it, they couldn't have been insulted; yet you, overridingly, did not want anyone to know that you were an "addict."

That's what we call "false pride," and false pride will get you into a lot of trouble. That same false pride is getting you into trouble with your wife and preventing you from bringing her in here so you can both get some help.

What would have been so terrible about telling her you needed that meeting, that you needed to share the experience with people who would understand? False pride stopped you. It seems like you didn't want to be "that bad," whatever that means. And as a result, you had an uncomfortable day.

Jim: Well, that's all true. You know that I still have trouble telling people. It's easier for me to introduce myself in meetings and say that I'm an addict, but in my personal and professional life I hate it. That false pride you're talking about probably does apply to me. But what do I do about it?

Therapist: If you don't think it's serving a purpose any more, you might let it go. And you could take a concrete step to letting it go by bringing your wife in here.

Jim: Okay, okay, I'll talk to her, and if she's willing

. . . no, I'm sure if I ask her to she'll come, she'll be nervous but she'll come . . .

Therapist: Great. I think that will be helpful to both of you. Shall we plan to meet with her at our regular time next week unless I hear from you differently?

Jim: Sure.

Therapist: Now let's go back to that incident and see how you could have handled it differently. . . .

When his wife came in the following week she was indeed nervous, but she said she was relieved to be able to know a little more about what her husband was doing with his time. She had hoped that when he'd stopped doing drugs he would be home with her more and they could enjoy each other again, but instead he always seemed to be going to meetings. We agreed to have four sessions and then recontract on how many to do from there. At the third session his wife, "Kate," said,

Kate: Well, I went to my first Al-Anon meeting this week and I liked it. If your AA and CA meetings are as good as that Al-Anon meeting, I can see why you go. Those people are so supportive and they seem to really understand.

Jim: Do you mean that? You mean it was good for you? But you didn't tell me you were going.

Kate: I didn't know till the last minute that I was, but Joanne had suggested I try it, and I decided to be spontaneous for once and try it. Like she said, I didn't have much to lose.

And another thing. I want to keep coming here for a while. I didn't tell you about going for another reason. When I felt so good after, I didn't know how to tell you. I realized that somewhere along the line we've stopped talking, and I think we need to start again. Maybe we can learn how here. [She takes a deep breath] That was hard to say, but I did it!

We recontracted for eight more sessions together and continued our work. During the sessions Jim and Kate were able to share a lot of their fears and hopes with each other and were also able to be more and more supportive of each other's recovery programs. Each reported being happier individually and a lot happier as a couple. At session ten of our working together, we talked about where to go in two more weeks. Did they want to continue their couple's work or begin to terminate?

Kate: If we can afford it, I want to keep coming. I can't believe all we've learned so far.

Jim: I agree, but money is a problem.

Kate: Oh, come on; money isn't really such a big problem. You've paid off all your drug debts. We've been managing for the last couple of months.

Jim: That's true.

Therapist: What's your reluctance besides the money?

Jim: Everything's changing so fast. I know it's all for the good, it's just going so fast. I'd almost like to take a break to let us get more comfortable with what we've got and then come in in a few weeks with the problems that come up. I don't want to learn anything else new for now. I've got enough to practice right now.

Therapist: That may be a valid point. How do you feel about that, Kate?

Kate: I feel like we need the support. I can see just practicing what we've gotten so far and not learning anything new for a few weeks, but I still think we need to come in here for support and pointers.

Jim: You mean you're willing to? You don't mind?

Therapist:	Wait a minute, your hidden reluctance was trying to protect her?
Jim:	[Sheepishly] Yeah, I guess so . . . I know she has to take care of herself. I guess I slipped there. I guess we do need your help. Sure, let's keep coming.

This is an example of a highly motivated couple who learned a lot about themselves and each other. After about a year they would occasionally come in for what we call "tune-up" sessions, but overall they are functioning quite well and are much happier than they'd thought they could be. They are still going to their meetings (AA, CA, and Al-Anon). At this time they are thinking of starting a family; Kate had said, "I didn't ever think he would be mature enough to be a father. Now I'm looking forward to seeing how good a father he'll be."

Jim was also amazed at how his wife "came through with such flying colors." As so often happens with couples affected by the disease of addiction, a lot of rescuing and saving goes on, each tries to second-guess and help the other person. Usually the straight member does that more than the using member, but then when the using member gets clean he often starts that kind of behavior because he is trying to make up for lost time—lost time when he was too stoned to know that she might have some needs too. That kind of behavior is referred to as co-dependency. The only way for the couple to change it is to start verbally expressing their needs until each one gets to a point where he/she is taking care of him/herself and not the other, trusting that the other person can take care of him or herself just fine and will ask for help when it is needed. Couple's counseling and Al-Anon are very helpful in uncovering those kinds of patterns and in finding new ways to deal with them.

GROUP THERAPY

Group therapy can be a very powerful and effective form of treatment. I co-facilitate recovery groups for people who have made a commitment to being clean and sober, and who are

actively working in a twelve step program. I also try to use a
male-female team so everyone in the group gets to deal with their
problems with both sexes. I like using a co-facilitator because it
allows me to keep my distance and perspective. I don't have to
do all the work; he shares it, and we can take turns—one of us
sits back for a time to watch the process, and the other listens
more for content. I enjoy the work more when I am part of a
good team. Whenever possible, I use a co-leader who is himself
recovering so we can share different perspectives with the members.

The group is a place where people can air any problems they
are having with living clean and sober, and get feedback and
suggestions from other people who are experiencing similar situations. It is very supportive and confrontive at the same time,
and people make a lot of progress by relating to other people in
the group who share similar problems. A successful recovery
group (like all other kinds of groups) comes to have an identity
of its own; it has life each time the group meets and the members
share their experiences. Here is an example of a group interaction:

Dana: I couldn't believe what happened this weekend.
          Remember I said that my best friend was getting
          married and I was going down to L.A. for the
          wedding? Well I did, and another good friend of
          mine, Elizabeth, was there. Well, old Elizabeth
          came up to me right off the bat, and before she
          could even say hello she said, "Got some good
          coke?" I told her I had stopped and she said, "But
          why?" I told her I had had a problem with it and
          she said, "But couldn't you have brought some for
          us? We didn't stop, and you always had the best
          stuff. That wasn't very considerate."

          I didn't know what to say, I was floored, the
          woman hadn't even said hello to me yet. I guess I
          looked pretty shocked or something, because she
          said, "Don't worry, I was only kidding." But then
          she walked away from me.

Later she came up and offered to buy me a drink. She said, "You looked upset before and I didn't mean to upset you. Let's have a couple of drinks and catch up on what's been happening." I went to the bar with her and ordered a Perrier and she said, in a very audible tone of voice, "Don't tell me you stopped drinking too." Well you can imagine—at that point I didn't know whether to throw the Perrier in her face, explain about addiction, or what . . . so I just said, "I sure did and I feel great."

Well, it took her no time at all to find someone she could have more fun with the way we always used to have fun. She invited a few other people who I didn't know to join us at the table, and I got pretty much shut out of the conversation and left. I don't seem to like bars very much anymore. But the whole wedding was like that. These were friends I used to use with, and I found out we didn't have much in common anymore. It was pretty sad, really. I could feel that after I got over the anger and embarrassment and decided that I was actually doing fine and wasn't going to be hurt by Elizabeth's opinions.

Gerry: Dana, you did great. I'm glad you weren't tempted to use. I think I would have told her off myself. You were real calm about it. God, I hate those kinds of experiences where, just because you're finally getting your life together, some schmuck who thinks he knows what he's doing comes up to you and acts like you're the freak. Being healthy sure puts you in a minority sometimes.

Therapist 1: That's true. But the longer you're clean, the more people you'll meet who are also in that new-found minority of yours.

Sherry: Well, sometimes I wish I'd meet them already. It gets pretty lonely out here being clean and sober and alone.

Bill: Yeah! Now when I go to a party and everyone's getting loaded, I don't even stay. They don't realize what little sense they are making. It's not fun anymore. Dana, I think you handled that situation well. Elizabeth sounds like she's pretty out there. I hope she didn't hurt you by how she treated you.

Dana: Thanks, Greg. Yeah, it hurt at first, but then I took a step backwards, something I couldn't have done if I'd been using, and I took another look at the situation; I felt like she was the one losing out, thinking she was so cool, surrounding herself with all these people and getting loaded. I was just upset that for a long time I was one of those people. So I'm pretty grateful not to be there anymore. And if that's the price I pay for being grateful, it's worth it. I like being able to wake up when the alarm goes off and feel clearheaded and know I can handle the day and I'll be at work on time rather than being foggy from being up most of the night snorting cocaine and looking for just one more line to help me get up; no thank you. I'd rather be a little ostracized at weddings and social gatherings than be part of that "in crowd" anymore.

Therapist 1: It sounds like it was a positive experience for you after all.

Dana: Yeah, it was. I guess I wanted to know if I handled it well. And you're telling me I did. Thanks, I just needed to make sure I did the right thing.

Sherry: Sometimes when I think someone is going to be as big an asshole as your friend Elizabeth was, I just say, "No, I don't have any" to requests for cocaine, and for a drink I say, "I just don't feel like it," or "No thank you." Then they can't make a big deal out of it. But I admire your candidness. I can't always be like that because I hate the consequences when people look at you like you're a freak.

Robby: Well, I just keep my baseball bat handy and bop them over the head when they're being an asshole. No, don't worry, I'm only kidding, but I sure feel like doing that sometimes.

Therapist 2: What do you do with those feelings?

Robby: I fantasize what I would do if I could and then I laugh at my absurdness in response to their absurdness, and then I know I'm still pretty crazy and I go to my meetings or call someone from this group and talk. It's been helpful having this group. I'm beginning to look forward to it during the week. It's a place I can speak my mind and my soul and be understood. And I thank you all for that.

Dana: Yeah, he's right. I thought down there of being able to come in today and talk about this. And I really looked forward to it. It's so important to be understood.

Groups can provide a safe atmosphere for learning with others how to cope with a new lifestyle. Most people in the groups I lead and co-facilitate have never been straight as adults. So they need to learn how to do it—how to be clean and sober every day and how to interact in social, business, and personal situations without the crutch of drugs. It is a new and exciting time for group members.

The co-therapists are there to make sure the group process is as honest and caring as possible, and to make sure that even the quiet members get their share. We try to make the group as egalitarian as possible; basically, we let the members bring up issues they want to talk about. During the life of the group we want them to do more and more of the work of running the group. We see them setting the focus and we keep track of the process, encouraging them to take over that role more so they know how to be effective group members by the time the group terminates.

LOOKING AT TRIGGERS FOR DRUG USE

Addiction is a relapsable, chronic, and often terminal disease. Although using is usually far from a person's mind during the middle stage of recovery, the possibility always exists. Because of this omnipresent reality, I ask clients to look at upcoming events that might, in the past, have triggered drug use as a way for them to cope or "go away" from the realities of the situation. Then we come up with alternative ways to respond so they don't have to escape through drugs.

It is indeed true that addicts use because they are addicts; however, anticipating an emotional event, planning for it, working the twelve steps, and perhaps going to a few extra meetings can be helpful. An addict can do some footwork to help assure staying clean, and that's what we do when we examine potential triggers. A trigger is a vulnerable situation; since addicts have dealt with vulnerable times for years by doing drugs, it's helpful to come up with some other options and possibilities so they can minimize that old tried and true but dysfunctional option.

A trigger may be a real event, or an anniversary of a real event. The unconscious is very powerful. Often we feel "funny"— depressed, sad, irritable, jittery, or extra nervous—for no apparent reason. Yet, when we look back, we find it is the anniversary of something traumatic, such as a parent's death, a rape, or a difficult divorce. Here's an example:

Terry: You know, it's strange; I've been feeling so good lately and pretty confident that I can handle what comes up in my life—well, not that I can handle the whole thing, but that between me and my higher power it'll be okay. But the last few days I've had this impending sense of doom. Like I want to run and hide. I do, I feel like running away. I think this is how I would feel before I started on a big run, or before I'd go traveling for a while. I don't quite understand it, and it's getting me a little worried.

I know you're going to tell me to go to a couple of extra meetings this week, and I plan on doing that, but this almost aching sense of doom . . . It's new for me to be feeling when I'm straight. I thought this would go away when I got clean.

Therapist: Not all your problems go away when you get clean. In fact, that's when you get to face them all. They haven't disappeared, you just get to deal with them clearheadedly and you get the help of your higher power, something you didn't have before.

It sounds like what you're feeling may be a symptom of what I call "the anniversary concept."

Terry: The what?

Therapist: The anniversary concept. Sometimes our unconscious reminds us on a subliminal level of something that happened a long time ago. We are not aware of it on a conscious level today, but somehow, at the time of year it originally happened, our brain triggers the same kind of emotions that occurred then. It could be something that happened last year, five years ago, ten years ago, or even twenty years ago. But when we have unfinished business, it tends to crop up. For instance, grieving is an emotion that we often have left unfinished.

When the anniversary triggers old emotions, you get another chance to deal with unfinished business. It's another chance your unconscious is giving you to heal yourself of old hurts.

Can you think of anything that happened at this time of year in your life that may have really set off some strong emotions that seem to be cropping up now saying, "Deal with me!"

Terry: I'm trying to think, but it's weird, all I want to do is leave. I have this incredible desire to leave right now.

Therapist: When have you ever needed to leave this urgently before?

Terry: I don't know.

Therapist: Sort back in your mind through the years and see if you can come up with anything.

Terry: [Looking upset] Oh my God! You won't believe this.

Therapist: Try me.

Terry: About thirteen years ago my brother died.

Therapist: You never told me you had a brother.

Terry: I didn't? Actually, that's not so surprising. I try not to think about it.

Therapist: It seems like you're thinking about it now. We may as well check it out, if you're willing.

Terry: I guess I'd better. I'm realizing that this is the time of year I always go away. Boy, have I hooked up with some characters, anyone I meet who's traveling anywhere. I leave San Francisco for a few weeks or even a couple of months and go away. Maybe if I look at this again—again? What am I saying? I've always avoided remembering my brother's death. It's been too painful. I hope there's plenty of tissues in that box.

Therapist: If there aren't I know there's plenty of toilet paper, so if you don't mind . . .

Terry: [Little laugh] No, and besides who am I to be overly proud? I can even use my shirtsleeve if it comes to that.

Therapist: Is this the time of year your brother died?

Terry: What's today's date?

Therapist: August 1.

Terry: That's incredible. He died August 3, 1971. You're not kidding about the old unconscious being powerful. I never associated all my crazy times with him dying.

Therapist: Can you talk about it?

Terry: I think I better. Only it's real hard. See, my brother drowned and I . . . I . . . I was supposed to be watching him. And I had been, I really had been. I was a pretty good big sister. I was three years older than him. We had gone down to the quarry where all the kids hung out during the summer. And my Mom had told me, as we left, to watch out for my brother. She always told me to watch out for him, and I usually did. Only, only, that day, oh shit, this is harder than I thought. [She begins to cry]

Therapist: You're doing fine. If you need to stop for a minute, go right ahead. This does sound hard to recall, but I bet you've needed to let this one go for a long time.

Terry: [She cries harder] I have, but I was always afraid to tell anyone. I feel so responsible. I didn't think anyone could still like me if they knew the whole story.

Therapist: Unless you held his head under the water and killed him, I think you're probably free of a lot of the responsibility you've taken on over the years. And from what I know of you, I don't think you could have done that to your brother.

Terry: [Looking up from her tears and tissue] You sure do have a way with words. Of course I didn't hold his head under water, but I did go off with my friends for a while, and I left him with his friends.

Therapist: Go on.

Terry: Well, like I said, I did leave him alone.

Therapist: Alone or with his friends?

Terry: With his friends. There were plenty of other people around. I never thought it was a dangerous situation, or I wouldn't have done it. I loved my little brother.

Therapist: I believe you. I'm sure you never would have purposely endangered him. You said the quarry was a place all the kids used to hang out, so it was obviously pretty safe.

Terry: And my brother was a good swimmer. A very strong swimmer.

Therapist: What happened?

Terry: This is the hard part.

Therapist: I know it is. But I honestly think it's better off said outside your body then left screaming at you inside. You've beat yourself black and blue with this one long enough. Let's try to get it out and see if it's less painful to you then. I'm pretty sure it will be. Willing to go at it a little more?

Terry: [Almost inaudibly] Yes. Well, my friends were going to drink some beer. One of the guys had stashed some beer up in the trees and a few of us were going to have a beer or two. See, that's where my drug use started. Actually, that was my first time invited to join the older kids for a beer, and I was feeling pretty big and important. But I even stopped long enough to find my brother and tell him I was going to go; and he knew what that meant.

My brother gave me kind of a crooked smile [more tears]. I'll never forget his expression, he knew I was going to do something I wasn't supposed to and he was kind of giving his approval. I could tell. We were so close that I knew he wouldn't tell Mom, and he didn't mind my going. I told him I'd be back in about a half hour, which I fully intended on being. He gave me a half pat, half shove on my back and said, "See you later, Sis." And I left. [She sits looking down into her lap, looking far away]

Therapist: You're doing fine. It sounds like you and your brother were very close. This had to have been very painful for you, and it still is. I'm here with you. You're not alone with this anymore. Can you keep going?

Terry: [Looks up and starts crying] Why did he have to do it? Why?

Therapist: Why did he have to do what?

Terry: Jump off the rocks. Jump—no, that wasn't enough. He dove off, they say. You see, the quarry had some rock cliffs left on one side. And the kids would dive off them . . . I always hated watching. I was afraid one of them would . . . would . . . would not dive out far enough and crack his head open. There were some angles that were more difficult than the rest.

My brother knew how scared I was of the cliffs. And that's why I feel so responsible. If I had been there, I might have stopped him. He usually listened to me. But I figured because I went off and was doing a "no-no" with my friends, drinking beer, that gave him permission to do what he wasn't supposed to do—dive off the cliffs. And he had to go off the more dangerous ones. Goddamn it, why wasn't I there to stop him! [She sobs openly]

Therapist: [I go over and put my arms around her as she cries] It's okay. Let it out, let it out. [She subsides] How do you know you could have stopped him? How many other kids dove off those cliffs and were okay? Were you supposed to watch him every minute of every summer so he never dove off those cliffs? Could you have? It sounds like he was a pretty adventurous kid, and you said he was a strong swimmer. It's not your fault. He dove and, if anything, it sounds like he knew very well how you felt about him doing that. And I'll bet that wasn't the first time he dove off them.

Terry: All that you're saying is true. He used to dive off the cliffs whenever he could. He used to tell me, "See, you don't have to be scared; nothing will happen." I'd hate it every time he scrambled up the rocks before I could catch him. And he was an adventurous kid. He really was. God, I miss him. I just wish he had dived out a little more instead of making my worst fear come true.

Therapist: Can you finish up this story?

Terry: Yeah, I better; the worst is almost over. God, I've never told anyone all this.

Therapist: Thanks for sharing it with me.

Terry: Thanks? What are you, morbid or something?

Therapist: See, you still have your sense of humor—you'll be fine.

Terry: Well, about halfway through the first beer I heard some shouting from below. The first few shouts I tried to wish into the "kids playing" category; but that didn't work and I immediately got this terrified feeling in my throat. I don't think it was so much intuition. I used to get that feeling a lot when I thought I might be responsible or involved in something wrong, and I was already wrong for drinking beer . . . anyway, we all started running back down the path towards the water.

I started looking around for my brother and I couldn't see him. And then I saw a group of kids in the water and they were dragging out another kid. I started yelling to see if someone had called an ambulance, no one had. One of my friends said he'd go call and the rest I see as me walking in a fog, but doing . . . doing whatever I could until the ambulance got there.

He had dived off and hit his head. Everyone thought it was just a scrape, because he continued into the water. Apparently, he must have turned his head to see something as he dove in and caught the left side on a jagged rock. It bruised his head and it must have knocked him out. And then he stayed under water too long and his friends thought he was only kidding and by the time they started yelling at him to surface and realized he wasn't going to . . . anyway, they started diving in and got him. I tried to make him comfortable. I held him in my arms, but he was so limp. None of us knew mouth to mouth resuscitation.

And I don't know if it even would have helped . . . He died on the way to the hospital. I wish he hadn't died. I really do. That little shit, I wanted him to be my lifelong brother and he had to be adventurous. Shit. Goddamn it!

Therapist: You must have been so upset.

Terry: Actually, I was in a kind of fog. I don't think the fog ever completely lifted till I got clean. I was in such shock at the time that our family doctor prescribed Valiums to relax me. And I felt so guilty for not stopping him, for being with my friends, that I started escaping more and more from our family home to my friends, and my friends became the kids who drank and did other drugs regularly.

You know, I never thought of it, but my parents really lost two kids that day.

Therapist: You mean one died and they lost the other to drugs?

Terry: Yeah.

Therapist: That's a good point. And now they may be lucky enough to get one back.

Terry: Not so fast. I still have a hard time with them.

Therapist: I know. And I'm not pushing you. We'll deal with that a little later. I have a feeling that when you can let yourself off the hook for your brother's death, you may have a lot easier time relating to them. I'll also bet that this is a very hard time of year for them, too.

Getting back to August 3, 1971—how did your parents react?

Terry: They never actually accused me. They asked me what

happened and I told them what people had told me.
I told them I was off with my friends for a few
minutes and my Mom shot me this look—I know it
wasn't accusatory; it was more like, "You know you
weren't supposed to do that." And that was all. We
all walked around like barely functioning zombies for
a long time. Occasionally, Mom cried. But my dad
is the strong, silent type, he never talked. This may
sound crazy, but we have rarely talked about my
brother. Occasionally, my mom and I will, but my
dad—he'll walk out of the room. I think it still hurts
us all a lot.

. . . You may be right about my parents having a
hard time right now. Maybe it's time we talked this
one out? Do you think I could do that?

Therapist: Do what?

Terry: Talk to them about this?

Therapist: About how you've felt all these years?

Terry: I guess that's what I mean.

Therapist: What would stop you?

Terry: Nothing. Just our old family tradition of silence.

Therapist: Is it time to break that tradition?

Terry: I think it is for me.

Therapist: Do you think they're ready?

Terry: I don't know. We've been talking a little more since
I've gotten clean, but this is a Biggie—with a capital B.

Therapist: What's the worst that could happen?

Terry: My father wouldn't want to hear.

Therapist: And what could you do?

Terry: Ask him to please try and stay.

Therapist: And if he still couldn't stay and talk?

Terry: Say the serenity prayer and talk with my mom.

Therapist: Any idea how you might feel?

Terry: Relieved. I definitely feel a lot better than when I walked in here today.

Therapist: You look a lot better. Your cheeks have some color in them now. What did you learn from this one?

Terry: Hmm . . . that I don't have to run away any more. I didn't kill my brother.

Therapist: He was the one who, knowing it could be dangerous, dove off those cliffs.

Terry: And like you said, I could have been there and watched the whole thing and I might not have been able to stop him even if I wasn't off drinking beer and had been there the whole time.

Therapist: That's true.

Terry: Then I don't have to go off and go away any more, at least not about this one. I think I've learned something else.

Therapist: What's that?

Terry: I can deal with reality and it won't kill me.

Therapist: Or anyone else?

Terry: Or anyone else.

Therapist: How are you feeling now?

Terry: Much better, thank you.

Therapist: Good, because we are going over and I'll have another session in a few minutes. Are you okay till next time?

Terry: I think so.

Therapist: This has been a heavy session. Remember, you can call me if you need to talk before our next session.

Terry: If I feel the urge to call my folks, I might need your help before or after I call.

Therapist: Please feel free to call. I'll be happy to help.

Terry: Thanks a lot. This was a really good session.

Therapist: You're very welcome. And thank you for trusting me enough to share all that with me. I know it was hard for you.

Terry: It was, but I feel a lot better.

Therapist: See you soon.

Terry: Have a good week.

Therapist: You too.

Terry had associated her brother's death with the need to escape at this time every year. When she left, I felt pretty sure that she was not going to have to keep on trying to escape from that memory. She had opened up about her brother's death in a way that she never had before. I think she let go of a lot of guilt for his death during our session, and she won't have as much pain to deal with. In her sobriety she has found new ways to deal with pain, and one of those is to allow herself to feel some pain and know she'll survive.

She did talk to her parents, and she was able to get support from her mom and her dad. It turned out her dad had felt guilty for years because he had been such a workaholic during the time the kids were growing up that he had felt he hardly knew his son; he felt he hadn't spent enough time with him teaching him what was right and wrong and what was dangerous. Terry was very surprised that her dad opened up to her; I suggested that the family had all been lost to each other long enough; that everyone had needed each other for a long time, but just didn't know how to reach out. I congratulated my client on being the first one to reach out, and on not feeling a need to run away and escape to a new place. As a matter of fact, she made a visit home to her parents for a long weekend and they all went to her brother's grave and planted some fresh flowers. It seemed to be a new beginning for the family. I think we succeeded in getting rid of the power behind this particular trigger.

TALKING ABOUT "SLIPS"

Addicts do sometimes slip and use drugs again at various stages during their recoveries. For some reason, critical times seem to occur when a person has been clean four to six weeks, at five to seven months, and then again around eleven to thirteen months. I try to warn people as they are coming up to these critical times and get them to anticipate emotionally charged upcoming events, increase the number of meetings they are attending, and make sure they are working on their recovery program; most important, I point out to them when it looks like they are trying to "run the whole show" and maintain control over their lives rather than admit that their lives are unmanageable and they are powerless over drugs. That is step one in their program: They must always be aware that their lives are uncontrollable and unmanageable. Most slips occur when addicts begin to think that they are in the driver's seat and thereby push out the concept that there is something greater than they are running the show. At that point they fall back into addictive thinking, and are most vulnerable to a slip.

People find it difficult to come in and tell me they have used after they've been clean a while. This seems to be the case even though I tell them addiction is a relapsable disease in which they can almost count on slips, and that the most important thing is to come in, talk honestly about them, to let go of the slips, and get right back into a recovery program. After people slip, their affect is often so different from usual that I know something's up. From nonverbal hints I can deduce that they've used. I try to get them to tell me; if they can't, then I express what I'm feeling and perceiving. At these times they usually feel they have failed, they feel ashamed and guilty. I try to get them to stop beating themselves up with those feelings and use their energy more positively, to get back into recovery.

Here's a young man, "Gordon," who had stopped using cocaine for six months and then slipped during a business trip.

Gordon: So, how are you doing?

Therapist: Fine, thanks. Aren't I supposed to be asking you that question?

Gordon: [Formally] Actually, you are.

Therapist: So, how are you doing?

Gordon: [Curtly] Fine, just fine.

Therapist: You seem a little on edge today. Are you?

Gordon: Maybe. You know, I've been traveling a lot for my job. I've been traveling across the country and even went to Italy once in the last month.

Therapist: I know, it's been a hectic time for you.

Gordon: It sure has. It also feels a little strange, because I haven't been in here for a few weeks. I managed to see you that once when I was in town for three days in between trips, but after that I've only been in town for one or two days at a time . . . that's why I had to cancel our other appointments.

Therapist: That's what you had said on my machine.

Gordon: So you got the messages.

Therapist: Yes, thanks for letting me know.

Gordon: [Testily] I said I would.

Therapist: Why does it feel like you're jumpy and defensive today?

Gordon: Like I said, it's been a while.

Therapist: Hmm. Were you able to get to some meetings while you were on the road?

Gordon: [Angrily] Come on, give me a break. I was traveling on business.

Therapist: I'm aware of that, but before you left we had talked about how long you would be on the road and you copied down AA meetings you were going to attend while you were gone.

Gordon: Yes, I did, but I found that to be too inconvenient.

Therapist: Inconvenient? Your recovery was inconvenient? Wait a minute, what happened to your priorities in the last month?

Gordon: [Angrily] Look, I had a lot on my mind. I needed to concentrate on business.

Therapist: Hold on a second, since when does concentrating on business preclude your recovery program?

Gordon: It doesn't preclude it, I just put it on the back burner for a few weeks. It's not that serious. Get off my case.

Therapist: Am I on your case? Somehow, this session feels strange to me. It feels like we're fighting about something that's not out in the open yet. Would you like to walk out of the room and come in again, and we can try this a little differently? We're both getting caught up in something and I think it's your addictive thinking at work again. I'm going to take a deep breath and slow down here and detach myself a little. [I take a deep breath, sit back, take another deep breath] Ah, that's better. So how are you doing?

Gordon: Lousy.

Therapist: That's better. Why?

Gordon: [With a half smile] Better that I'm doing lousy?

Therapist: No, I meant better that you're being more honest. Want to tell me what happened when you put your recovery on the back burner?

Gordon: It seems like you know already.

Therapist: Know what?

Gordon: I used a couple of times when I was over in Italy.

Therapist: Used?

Gordon: Don't act so surprised.

Therapist: It's not such a surprise, so much as I'm trying to find out what you used, how much, when, where?

Gordon: Is it even so important?

Therapist: The facts in and of themselves, are not so important. What is important, is that you can be honest about it.

Gordon: Oh. And then?

Therapist: Then we can reexamine your recovery program, see what's missing, and see where you go from here. Right off the bat what seems to be missing is a priority.

Gordon: I know you're going to say that back-burner status isn't high enough.

Therapist: And what do you say about that?

Gordon: You're probably right.

Therapist: Probably?

Gordon: Okay, it's not enough.

Therapist: Are you just saying that to please me, or because you believe it?

Gordon: No, I believe it. I'm just a little ashamed of myself, so I'm giving you a hard time.

Therapist: Well, why don't you be nicer to you, and then you can be nicer to me?

Gordon: But I'm upset about it. I was doing so well, six months without a slip. And then all of a sudden I'm at square one again.

Therapist: I can understand your being upset, but you're not at square one again.

Gordon: I'm not? How do you figure that?

Therapist: At square one you'd be asking me about how you could socially use cocaine and continue to socially drink. I hope you are still convinced that you have to be abstinent.

Gordon: I see what you mean. But to tell you the truth, it takes a lot of time to stay clean. It's a lot to go to meetings, come here, always be explaining myself . . .

Therapist: Are you saying you'd rather use again? Doing drugs wasn't time consuming? I seem to recall you saying that you were staying up most nights until the wee hours snorting cocaine, and that you were barely functional during the day. Excuse me, but could you please point out to me how being clean and sober and functioning all day is "more time consuming"?

Gordon: [Laughs] You caught me again. You sure are good at that. I guess that's my crazy thinking again.

Therapist: What's it going to be?

Gordon: I don't know, I honestly don't. I did like how I was feeling when I was clean and sober and working my recovery program, but it was difficult when I was on the road, especially when I was in Italy. Drinking is such a part of their day that business deals were always being closed with some wine, or wine at dinner and wine at lunch. I just broke down at some point in all those offerings and said "Yes, thank you" instead of "No, thank you." That's all it was, a few glasses of wine. I didn't get into any cocaine there or in the three days I've been back.

Therapist: I ask you again; what's it going to be from here?

Gordon: I'd like to be able to drink occasionally.

Therapist: I'm sure you would, but . . . ?

Gordon: I know I can't. I felt lousy after I drank the wine, and I've felt lousy and scared ever since. That's why I was jumping all over you when I first came in. I am sorry for doing that.

Therapist: Thank you for the apology. I appreciate you recognizing that so quickly. But where do you want to go from here?

Gordon: [Glancing at watch] I think I'll have time to get some dinner at that restaurant around the corner and then I'd better go to an 8 P.M. AA meeting.

Therapist: Is that something you want to do for you?

Gordon: Yes. It is. I guess I really don't want to start using again; otherwise, I would have canceled my appointment today.

Therapist: Did you consider that?

Gordon: I sure did. But I knew that was just too nuts. I figured coming to see you might be a positive influence on me.

Therapist: And has it been?

Gordon: Obviously. I'm going to a meeting tonight. How many meetings do you think I should make this week?

Therapist: You've had six months of experience with this, what do you think?

Gordon: Probably at least five. Do you have another hour open later in the week?

Therapist: As a matter of fact, I do, on Thursday afternoon at four.

Gordon: Good. I'll be here.

Therapist: See you then.

Gordon had fidgeted and acted testy from the moment he walked into my office, and I'd known something was wrong from the start. Often, with addicts, a therapist's first intuition about what's going wrong is that the person has used. I try to consider other options, but I must say that's usually my first idea unless I know of some impending crisis such as losing a job or breaking up with a girlfriend. I can be pretty sure when clients are unusually defensive or short with me that they've slipped and are feeling badly about themselves for having used again. It seems to be a fairly common reaction for them to be defensive and angry with the therapist—what Freud would call projection, and what I see as partly an angry stance, saying, "You didn't do enough for me. See, I'm not cured yet"; or "See, you had faith in me and I believed you, but I am really as hopeless as I thought I was."

I try to deemphasize the slip itself and reroute the person back into a more successful recovery program. In the next few sessions, we will examine what Gordon had been feeling about himself when he refused the offers of wine in Italy. I would also want to know what he was telling himself as he was refusing, when he stopped refusing, and when he started again. He seems to know that what happened is largely his addictive thinking taking over again. There is also a strong connection with his being on temporary hold from recovery—not seeing me and not going to meetings—and slipping. This experience should reinforce his notion about what he has to do to stay clean and sober. His commitment to go to five meetings in the ensuing week and to see me for an extra session indicated that he is well on his way.

A slip does not have to develop into a run. People can catch themselves and get back on the right track. I try to reframe their negative perspective into a positive option so they can't stay stuck beating themselves up with their "error," but rather can use that energy therapeutically in a more positive way.

SUPPORT FOR REMAINING CLEAN

I give the people I work with a lot of support for remaining clean throughout their recovery process. Periodically, we review what is different in their lives and how they think the absence of drugs has affected them. At the beginning of their recovery program, I ask them to keep a journal and record all their progress so they can look back and read about their recovery. Sometimes memory lets pain and small steps to progress fade as time moves on, so I want them to have an account of how they have changed, how they felt, and what new behaviors they are learning.

It is usually hard for people to take compliments at first, but they learn; usually, after they have learned to give themselves compliments, they can accept compliments from others. Whenever I say something supportive, I also try to get them to acknowledge something they are pleased with in themselves. At times they are afraid they will get too egotistical, but I reassure them that if I ever see their ego walking into the room first and them following, I'll be sure to tell them; but until then, they can acknowledge themselves to their heart's content.

Addicts are usually so down on themselves by the time they reach a therapist's office that I rarely have a problem with people being too self-inflated, unless it's along the lines of false pride. False pride usually shows up in bragging about how much coke they've done or dealt, and how "fucked-up" they've become. I'm not impressed by or interested in these things, and I let them know it.

Most people appreciate being rerouted to a different conversational level; but some who have operated at that plane for a long time find it difficult to talk about anything else. They've wowed people for a long time with their drug talk, and when they meet someone who's not impressed, they don't know quite what to do. But that's usually in early treatment sessions when their lives still revolve around drugs. Usually, by the middle stage of treatment, they have shed those layers of false pride and are building themselves up as human beings again. They are building new lives and are more eager to talk about their new lives than their old drug lives.

Therapist: You look happy today.

Jeff: I am. I got my six-month chip at CA last night.

Therapist: Congratulations! That's right, I had forgotten you were getting that this week. How does it feel?

Jeff: Pretty incredible. I sure didn't think I'd see this day when you started talking to me about going to AA and CA seven months ago. It took me a while to get into it. Remember, I was slip-sliding away for a while there till you caught me and said I had two more weeks to decide if I was going to be in recovery or you wouldn't see me anymore. Then I listened up fast.

Therapist: Thanks for the compliment. But really, you did the work, I could have said to you, "It's two more sessions and you need to decide if you want to be in recovery or not," and you could have said, "Later" to me; in fact, many people have done just that. So please, you deserve the credit for being clean. I'm not doing it for you, and I didn't make you do it six months ago. It's you going to all the meetings, it's you refusing drugs, it's you creating a new lifestyle for yourself. That's all you and your higher power. And I think you're doing great!

Jeff: Do you really think so?

Therapist: Are you fishing for a compliment or what?

Jeff: [Laughs] I guess I was.

Therapist: I tell you what, if you don't have anything pressing you need to talk about, why don't you start talking about all the changes you've experienced in your life in these last six months, and then I'll tell you about some of the positive changes I see.

Jeff: Okay, that sounds like fun. Sure, I didn't have that much else to talk about. I am kind of pumped up about getting my chip. Like I said, I sure never thought I'd see this day six months ago. That's a big change right there. Plus, when I tried to envision it, I sure didn't see myself feeling this good or enjoying myself and life so much. I saw being straight as boring, definitely boring to the max. And it's not at all.

Therapist: Would you like to start there?

Jeff: Where?

Therapist: How unboring life is?

Jeff: It's really not boring. I'm still going to three or four meetings a week, and that alone keeps me pretty busy. And I almost always learn something there. It is amazing. Someone always says something that I can relate to or learn from. And you were right.

Therapist: Me?

Jeff: You had told me a long time ago that learning could be fun. Remember when I was having trouble accepting that I had to change so much?

Therapist: I sure do.

Jeff: You suggested that if change scared me so much, I should look at the situation differently. You reminded me that I had been a very good student in school, that I had liked learning and doing well all those years in school, and you suggested that I view my recovery as a degree in life and learn all I could. You told me to forget about changing and just concentrate on learning. And it worked. I learned new ways of being, and by learning them I could try them out. For some crazy reason that was an easier thing for me to do than thinking about making a lot of changes. I ended up changing a lot, but it was by learning and being confident in what I was learning.

Therapist: I'm glad that worked for you. The end result is a much happier and healthier person than the one who first walked into this office seven months ago.

Jeff: I feel like a huge load has been lifted off my back, only I know I have to watch it because I can still see it in the corner of my eye; that load is addiction and it's off my back, but it's still within sight. I realize now that I have to keep it within sight so I can stay clean, knowing the other option of using is close to my side all the time. I don't feel as afraid of that as

I used to; it feels more like a healthy respect for that possibility.

Therapist: That sounds like a reasonable stance. You started talking about how unboring life is. Would you go back to that?

Jeff: I'm so busy that I have to remember to schedule in quiet, down time to regroup and reenergize so I don't spin out and have a non-drug case of stimulation overload. I do exercise three times a week. I make it a practice to eat well and don't eat junk food more than once or twice a week. And all that takes time. It's been good to see my body get in shape. I have a long way to go, but I'm on the road. I haven't had defined muscles like these in my arms since I was on the gymnastics team in high school, and that's a long time ago.

Besides doing all these things, just living and being able to notice things in the world around me is fun. I can walk down a street now or even drive down a street and notice people, kids, flowers, houses, trees, and crazy people. I know all these things have been here all along, but when I was using I just didn't have the time or the energy to notice them. When I think back, my life was so grey-hazy-drug-fogged; it's a wonder I didn't get into an accident driving around noticing so few details. I'm thankful that I got my awareness back.

That's what I think is largely responsible for me saying life isn't boring. It's actually become quite fascinating to just be alive. Sometimes I feel like I've been given a gift of my senses back, and it's wonderful. Not every day, mind you, but overall, my life is much much better than it had been when I was using. I wouldn't trade this for that for anything!

Therapist: I really enjoy hearing you talk about the changes in your life. It makes me feel good for you. I know you are hurting so much less than when you first came in. You were so afraid then that you would feel like that forever and you were also so afraid of feeling anything differently that you were really stuck. And to see how unstuck you are now is very gratifying.

                        I'm so glad, for you, that you've stayed with all this and faced your fears in a way that was not impossible for you, and you've learned a new way of living. You've got some more to learn, but you now have some solid building blocks to add further learning to; I think it'll be easier to go forward from here because you can look back on all you've learned in the last six months, feel good about that, read in your journal where you were and where you are, and get some impetus from it to keep going.

                        How do you feel about yourself in terms of pride in yourself?

Jeff: Pride? That's a good question. I think that was lost there for a while, especially after you introduced me to the concept of false pride. I know I walked in here with what I thought of as pride, but I realized from what you said that it was false pride at best. I really had no pride in myself and hadn't for a long time. But I have it now. When I went up to get my six-month chip at the meeting, I was so proud, so proud and so grateful. I could feel my cheeks were all flushed and my posture was straight. I felt like I really earned that chip, honestly earned it.

Therapist: It's been quite an accomplishment for you. I remember a time when even if you had accomplished something, you didn't feel good enough to acknowledge it or feel any pride. When you stayed clean for a week for the first time, you didn't want to acknowledge that at all—in fact, you insisted on minimizing it. It's nice to see that progress in you.

Jeff: Progress is a good term. I've made a lot of progress in the last six months, and I plan on making a lot of progress in the next six months. Or at least I hope to continue. I don't want to get too cocky here.

Therapist: I don't see that as too cocky.

Jeff: That is something I need to learn more about— feeling good and not being too scared of becoming too egotistical. I want to feel good, but keep it in an appropriate perspective.

Therapist: There's time to learn that. We can talk about that some more right now if you feel like you've done enough review of the last six months.

I give people support all along the way for the progress they have made. One reason for this is to role model for them how to take note of positive accomplishments and progress, because my clients have often forgotten how or never knew in the first place. It's so important for people to feel good about themselves if they are going to remain clean and be happy; and self-recognition is a key to self-esteem building. In turn, good self-esteem is a key to feeling good about oneself.

When I feel that I've role-modeled enough encouragement and support, little by little I get them to give themselves more and more support and then I simply reinforce it. In this way I hope to minimize their dependence on me and have them incorporate giving support into what they do for themselves regularly.

BEGINNING TO LOOK AT HOW TO MAKE NEW FRIENDS AND HOW TO HAVE FUN

In order to stay clean and sober, many of the people I work with have to give up a lot of the friends they had used with. It's very difficult for a person new to recovery to be around people who are using or are high. Being around drugs can trigger their own usage, or at least ambivalence and uncomfortable feelings, like, "Why can't I?"

Sometimes, old using friends try to get the person to use again and "have some fun, a little won't hurt." They may mean well, but they just don't know that a little will hurt a lot. They do not know about the disease of addiction; and usually they don't want to know, because then they might have to look at themselves and they don't want to do that. Especially if it would imply a change in their lifestyles. It's too threatening for them, and because of that threatening factor, friends may have an unconscious investment in keeping all people around them hooked. So newly recovering addicts often find themselves without friends to do healthy, non-drug-related activities with.

During beginning phases of recovery, addicts usually feel so badly about themselves that they don't think they're worthy of friendship; and that dissuades them from going out and finding new friends. It takes a while for addicts to realize that not all people have fun by getting high. Often they're afraid that they'll be the odd one out, or that no one will understand. Thus a lot of recovering addicts begin to meet people through the meetings they go to a few times a week; eventually, they stay after meetings and, when they have the courage, strike up conversations with other people or others strike up conversations with them. Alcoholics Anonymous, Cocaine Anonymous, and Narcotics Anonymous offer various activities, such as dances, picnics, and trips. These are fairly safe places to meet people, because you know drugs will not be brought up in an uncomfortable way.

One woman who had been clean for about nine months said, "But it's beginning to feel like I'm involved in two worlds, AA and the real world, and I'd like them to be more integrated." She meant that in AA and CA she could be honest and trust people and reach out and know they would understand, but she was reluctant to try that out in the "real world." Why? "People can be so much meaner in the real world."

We looked at her response and talked about places at work where she might watch out for people who might not be mean. I reassured her that not all the nice people in this world are recovering addicts. "There are at least a few other people out there who are real nice too." She decided to watch people interacting in the cafeteria at work and see if she could observe any interactions that might be acceptable to her. In two weeks she reported that there were a few women who did seem to be on friendly terms and met for lunch a few times a week. In a few weeks she built up her courage and sat at the table with them. Within a few weeks she had a fairly comfortable rapport with them and looked forward to meeting them for lunch.

People who are just beginning to socialize also have to work through issues concerned with saying "No, thank you" to offers of drugs and alcohol. In most cases, if they comfortably and self-assuredly say, "No, thank you," they are not questioned or bothered and will be offered a soft drink instead. If they say "No, I'm an addict; I don't do drugs," and they say it with assurance, they may get a few curious questions, but not as many negative responses as they had expected when they were too scared to socialize and used their negative fantasies as blocks to even trying. One young man said, "I can't believe it; girls seem to really like that I don't do drugs and that I don't drink. I'm finding more girls want to go out with me now than ever before. I could have at least once date a night if I wanted. I guess they think I'm stable or something. But they seem to admire me instead of thinking I'm a freak, which is what I was afraid of for so long."

The realistic picture is that some people will be turned off and not want to pursue a relationship with an addict. That is a fact of life, but even more people probably won't care. I remind clients that you can't please all of the people all of the time, and we try to look at the brighter side of things. "Just look at how easily that relationship ended instead of your agonizing for months or years over whether it was right or not." And we laugh.

Of course, sometimes we can't brush it off that easily. If a person is truly hurt by the experience, we'll talk about the hurt.

It's important for addicts to realize they have not been rejected for who they are, but for one small piece of what they are; the rejector has rejected a label—"addict"—not the person's love; and the part that's hurting is the core, which the rejecter never even saw and perhaps never tried to see.

I try to get clients to see this as a prejudiced view and a prejudiced act. Then we can talk about prejudice and how it is based on a fear of the unknown. I want people to separate the hurt from themselves and see that "they" haven't really been rejected, their addiction has been rejected. And a person who hasn't been able to see any deeper than the label probably isn't worth knowing anyway. In most cases, as addicts become more comfortable with themselves and what they need to stay clean and sober, they are able to discuss that more easily and are in turn accepted by others more easily. Addicts can do anything anyone else can, except take drugs. When they realize this, they don't have much trouble finding friends.

In the first year of recovery, it has been suggested that single people remain single and not embark upon a serious relationship. Addicts need the time during that first year to devote to themselves, to their recovery, to learning and changing without the pulls of a relationship. The first year will be emotional enough without the emotional pulls of another person, though this does not preclude friendships, which can be very helpful to a person's growth. But the focus needs to remain on recovery for the first year. I try to get people to keep this perspective as they begin to seek new friendships and begin to round out their lives a little more.

Partly because of all the changes addicts go through in the first year of recovery, it is important that if significant others feel neglected or upset with these changes that they go to Al-Anon or Nar-Anon where they can learn to deal with the changes they are going through in response to and apart from their friend or partner. All involved need support, and it is available. If changes and compromises in old relationships are not made, people will revert back to old habits. Changes can be made more easily if they are accomplished within a climate of support and caring which new friends and meetings can provide.

GENERATING NEW OPTIONS FOR A DRUG-FREE LIFESTYLE

I work with my clients to generate new options for drug-free lifestyles from the first time they enter my office until they terminate treatment. During the initial phase of treatment our work focuses on detoxification and an introduction to the reality of staying drug free. During the middle stage of treatment, when we focus more on maintaining sobriety, they have some extra energy to begin to explore new ways of having fun. I say new because, while their focus in life had been getting, doing, and recovering from drugs, all "fun" was associated with getting high, so their repertoire of possibilities for fun without drugs has been largely depleted. One man, "Don," had stayed clean by going to work, going to meetings, and going home. He was a very shy man and had not been able to socialize after meetings.

Don: This is getting ridiculous. I know you keep saying being clean and sober is great, but I don't feel that yet. I do feel better than when I was using, and I have some money saved up, but I'm still feeling like I'm not having any fun and like I'm alone.

Therapist: That's a pretty realistic assessment of your situation. I don't know how you could feel anything but alone, because you are alone and so far you've held out your fear of people as an effective block towards meeting anyone new. People usually don't do things differently until the pay-offs for doing things the old ways don't work any more. Is that the point you're at? Or are the old pay-offs from loneliness still too hard to give up?

Don: When you put it that way, I guess I still find stabil-

232   /   ONE STEP OVER THE LINE

ity in my loneliness. But it's getting annoyingly
uncomfortable.

Therapist: That's an interesting way of putting it. I've never
heard that expression before, "annoyingly uncomfortable." What do you want to do about that?

Don: My problem is I don't know. I've always been such
a loner that I honestly have no idea what else I can
do.

Therapist: You want to try something different, that might be
fun?

Don: Yes.

Therapist: Okay, let's see if I have a bag in my closet. [I go over
to my closet] Good, here's one that'll do [I pick up
a lunch-size paper bag]

Don: Do for what?

Therapist: We're going to make a grab bag of options for you.

Don: Oh come on, give me a break.

Therapist: I am, believe me; I'm trying to give you a break.

Don: Sometimes you come up with some great ideas, but
sometimes . . .

Therapist: Hear me out. If after we try this you still want to
reject it, or if you come up with a better idea of your
own, great. If not, maybe you'll try it out. It's worked
for other people.

Don: Okay. What are you going to do?

Therapist: Not just me, we are going to do this part together.
Here's a piece of paper. I want you to write down
anything you can think of that has ever struck your
fancy, and that is feasible to do, that might be fun.

Don: Like what?

Therapist: Like going to a movie, like learning how to play tennis, like hiking, like joining a book club. I don't know what your taste is in these kinds of things, so you need to help.

Don: Okay, let's see. Riding my bike is one.

Therapist: Good, write it down. Then skip a line, because in the end you'll cut out all your options and throw them in the bag. Then whenever you want to do something you'll just shake up the bag and put your hand in and pull something out. If you don't feel like doing that one you can pull out another choice. Let's try to come up with fifteen to twenty things you could do.

Don: And you expect me to do this?

Therapist: Got any better ideas to get you doing something that might be fun?

Don: [Laughs] No, I have to admit that. All right, let's get to work. I've written down bike riding.

Therapist: What's something else you could do?

Don: I've always wanted to get a massage and I never did that.

Therapist: Well, what's stopping you? Now that you're not doing cocaine, you have some extra money.

Don: Okay, I'll write that down. And another thing is going up to Calistoga and having the whole works; that only costs $50, I hear, and I used to spend a lot more than that on a good night with cocaine. I could put that down as another option. Drive up to Calistoga and get a massage and a mud bath and the whole thing.

Therapist:	Speaking of drives, have you ever driven out Highway 1 towards Stinson Beach and Point Reyes? That's a very nice drive. And if you continue up Highway 1 towards Dillon Beach, there's a good oyster bar restaurant. It's a good day trip any time of year. The flowers are really pretty now and for the next few months.
Don:	No, I never did go that way. That sounds good. Let me write that down. I've also never gone whale watching, and I hear that's fun.
Therapist:	We've got five things already. Great. Keep going.
Don:	When I was little I used to go camping with my family. But I haven't done that in a long time. I don't think that would be fun doing alone, though . . .
Therapist:	I've gone camping alone and I really enjoyed it. I love being in the country, and when I had the time and nobody I knew wanted to go, I just went. I always met people along the way if I wanted to, and if I wanted to be alone I could be.
Don:	Well, if you can do it . . .
Therapist:	See if you can think of some things closer to home to do on an evening where you don't want to drive a lot.
Don:	A movie, or a concert.
Therapist:	How about going to a café on Clement Street and watching the people go by?
Don:	Like in Europe?
Therapist:	Yeah, but right in your own backyard.
Don:	Geez, we've got nine things already.
Therapist:	How about the dances sponsored by AA or CA? You

know, there is one every Saturday night at the Alano Club.

Don: I suppose, but you know how hard that kind of stuff is for me.

Therapist: I know, but it sounds like sitting at home alone is getting hard too.

Don: Yup. Hmm . . . What about bowling? Do people still do that?

Therapist: I think so.

Don: Good, now I have ten things I could do.

Therapist: If you would consider the dances, I think that would make eleven things. You'll see a lot of people who are familiar from meetings.

Don: Okay, okay I know you're right; it's just . . .

Therapist: It's just what?

Don: I can't really think of any more excuses, but I'm scared. Geez, that old fear . . . I just wish it would disappear.

Therapist: Wait a minute. It is disappearing at the rate you are letting it go.

Don: Huh?

Therapist: Look at all the progress you've made in the last few months. For each step you've made, you've let a little bit of your fears go.

Don: Oh, yeah. I have, haven't I? Okay, the Alano Club dance next!

Therapist: Keep going; you're on a roll now.

Don: I could watch TV. I know I do that a lot now, but it is an option, and if I pulled that out of the bag and I didn't feel like doing that I might be more likely to pull out another idea that might be more fun instead of just succumbing to the boob tube.

Therapist: Good reasoning.

Don: You know what else I'd really like to do?

Therapist: No. What?

Don: Join a health club so I could have the option of working out. And I used to really like volleyball. Maybe I can find one that has volleyball.

This is fun. I'm getting excited just thinking about all these things. I always feel so uncreative when I'm home in my apartment feeling like there's nothing to do.

Therapist: It's no wonder, with that attitude—feeling like there's nothing to do—it's hard to think of something when you're sure there's nothing.

Don: [Laughs] There's my old positive thinking at work again.

Therapist: How many options for fun do you have?

Don: Let's see, I'll count them—hey, there's fourteen already. Let's get a couple more and then I can add some more as I think of them.

Therapist: Okay, that sounds fine. What about tennis?

Don: That's okay, but I need to have someone to play with.

Therapist: Do you know anyone who plays that you could ask?

Don: Actually, I do. I know a few people at work and I've overheard a couple of people at meetings. Okay, I'll put that one down. It'll involve calling a few people, but I should be able to do that. And there's some outdoor courts by my house.

Tennis, that's fifteen. And maybe just calling someone for dinner. Did you hear that just flow out of my mouth? Me, scared and meek. Well, I can. I am capable of that. I *am* a loner, but I have had dinner with people. I don't even slobber too badly anymore. [We both laugh]

Therapist: It's nice to see you get your sense of humor back. It's been rather dormant for the past few weeks.

Don: If just thinking about doing fun things does this to me, just imagine what actually doing these fun things will do. Watch out!

Therapist: I think I can handle it; can you?

Don: Just try me. Let's see in a couple of weeks what Mr. Fun Guy is like.

Therapist: We're running out of time. Want to cut up the list and put it in your grab bag?

Don: When you first suggested this I thought it was the corniest idea I had ever heard. And corny is a nice way for me to put what I thought about it. But now it seems like a good idea. I sure had fun doing it.

Therapist: Sometimes corny things aren't half bad.

Don: Got a scissor?

Therapist: Right here.

[Don cuts up the list, puts the items in the bag, and twists the top of the bag shut.]

Don: See you next week.

Therapist: I'll be interested to hear how your grab bag works for you this week.

Don: Me too.

The old grab bag trick works for a lot of things. I've used it to generate ideas for having fun, for alternatives to using, for when they get sad, and so on. Some people never have to use the bag itself, just the exercise of coming up with so many options seems to plant the seed and they think of ideas without going to the grab bag. Some people really enjoy the grab bag and use it and add to it as they think of more things they could do. Don came back the next week and said he had gone to a funny movie, gone out to Point Reyes on the weekend, and had a tennis game planned for that evening before a meeting. His affect was much lighter than it had been the week before.

The middle stage of treatment is the longest. It begins when addicts are ready to look at life a little more broadly than just asking how they can stay clean for one day at a time. When they are a little more confident that sobriety is something they want, they can begin to look at other areas that begin to surface. They always need to be aware of the effects drug use has had on these other areas, and how to eliminate these effects and generate new options; this then becomes the main theme during the middle stage of treatment.

The middle stage can go on for months or years. It is over when either the client or the therapist begins to talk about termination, and both agree that it is an appropriate time to begin to terminate. I try to have six weeks to two months in which to terminate so we can review the progress made; plan for what it's going to be like without the set support of therapy sessions each week; and, if at all possible, have a couple of weeks where we spread the sessions to every other week so the person gets to feel what it's like without a therapy session each week. I always leave the door open for the person to return for tune-up sessions along the way; or, if large issues that need more time arise, people are welcome to return. This final stage of treatment is the topic of the next chapter.

12. Terminating Therapy

Because addiction is a chronic, relapsable disease, recovery is a life-long endeavor. But one-to-one therapy does not have to be a consistant part of a recovery program in order for a person to stay drug free. Individual therapy may be used once, or it may be needed at various times during a person's life.

Terminating treatment in and of itself can be a therapeutic process. There are no ground rules for termination, no set amount of time to say, "I've been in long enough, it's time to stop." Therefore the decision to terminate is an individual one. It is based on each person's progress in therapy, and ideally it is a mutual decision made by the client and the therapist.

I bring up the possibility of terminating when it seems to me the client has reached or achieved the goals outlined during the first two stages of treatment, and has been able to incorporate them into daily life. I also take into consideration how comfortable the client has become with the changes. The client needs to know that meeting the present goals is not a "cure," and should be familiar enough with the recovery process that the one-to-one therapeutic interactions each week are no longer necessary; the ongoing plan put in motion by both client and therapist should help assure continued success. Termination can be a very positive experience when the client and therapist both agree it's time.

When we begin to talk about the possibility of terminating our therapeutic relationship, I try to get clients to allow for six to eight weeks of terminating. Termination should not be an abrupt ending; it should be a process, so clients can get used to the idea that they will no longer be getting guaranteed support from a person they have come to rely on to be there when needed.

Even though, intellectually, clients usually feel ready to end treatment, they are usually not aware of the emotional changes terminating will cause; and they have not anticipated feelings of loss, abandonment, and fear, and more positive emotions such as independence and the ability to rely on others. This gamut of feelings and reactions is so common that therapists must warn people to anticipate them and work them through before terminating, so they are not caught unawares after an abrupt termination.

I also use some of this time to review all the progress that has been made. Clients need to go over all they have learned about themselves, their lives, the world around them, and the ways they fit into that world in a positive, healthy way. I am able to share my perceptions of how they have grown and learned and changed. I also share with clients what I've learned from them, and what working with them has been like for me. I have the client look at what it's been like working with me, and they share their ideas and perceptions about the therapeutic process. We use the last six weeks to two months to go over where we've been together, where they have been, what they've learned, and where they're going from here.

When we take the time to go over and finish up business, they can leave with positive feelings about the work we've done and with some direction for keeping it going with less formal supports. This will be very helpful to continued recovery. Endings are so difficult for most people that termination can actually be a very therapeutic way to teach someone how to end things positively and feel good about moving on.

So often people stay in the same place, unhappy or uncomfortable, but too scared and insecure, afraid of the unknown or of hurting someone's feelings, to move. So they stay stuck. By terminating over a period of time, people can see and feel, firsthand, that leaving, and endings do not have to be so painful. You always take something of what you've experienced with you; and when we go over what has been learned, clients get that sense of taking a lot with them in a very powerful way. After experiencing a positive ending process to formal treatment, it is usually easier for them to end other things when they need to do so.

Another important lesson to be learned from termination is

that endings do not have to be final. Many people seem to burn their bridges as they cross them. I leave the option open for further work. They are always welcome to come back at a later date, either for a visit or two over a specific issue, or for more long-term work if that need should arise. I view life as a series of onion peelings: every time you peel off a layer of onion, there is another layer underneath to be dealt with; and some will be dealt with more easily than others. People are welcome back when the onion peeling causes too many tears; and they are welcome to come back and share something good or joyous with me. I also do follow-up phone calls with people I have worked with. Usually, I call every six months or so to see how they are doing. It's nice for both of us to talk about the progress they have continued to make on their own. Sometimes, my calling is a way they can ask for help again because they have been unable to initiate contact themselves. More often, they are doing well and are happy to share their pride in their new lifestyle and how well they've been doing.

Sometimes people decide they are ready to terminate, and the therapist does not agree. When that happens I tell them how I feel about their quitting and why I don't think it's a good idea. I present evidence to back up my perceptions that they would be terminating prematurely. I listen to their ideas and perceptions and present, in turn, what I see as a less distorted picture of what is happening.

At times, they agree that they're being premature and decide to stay and work through whatever issues had begun to block their progress and make them want to avoid and flee instead of stay and face the fears and work them through. At other times, I am not able to get them to see what they are doing as I see it; then I have to deal with my own negative feelings. When that occurs I share my reactions with the client, but any leftover feelings that I think might be burdensome I share with a fellow professional or through Al-Anon and its principles of letting go of that which you can't control. I'm sure these leftover feelings are evidence that my "save the world" syndrome is still kicking around in the recesses of my brain. What I share and what I keep to myself during a difficult termination depends on what I think is therapeutic and what I think is too much rescuing. My therapeutic concerns for the clients' welfare get expressed, and those I can recognize as too much rescuing I have to deal with elsewhere.

When clients end before they are ready and the therapist allows it to happen without burdening the client with the therapist's ideas and perceptions, then the door is more open for them to return when they realize it was a premature ending. No "I told you so's" allowed here—although I have been tempted a couple of times. Instead, I laugh at myself and welcome the person back.

A GOOD TERMINATION

Let's take a detailed look at excerpts from a situation in which a client, "Bret," wants to terminate treatment and agrees to come for an eight-week termination process.

THE FIRST WEEK

Bret: While you were on vacation I had time to think about all that has happened in the last year and a half, and a lot has changed.

Therapist: I agree, you have changed a lot of things in your life.

Bret: Well, I was thinking that I might be able to use these two hours a week that we meet in different ways.

Therapist: What are you saying?

Bret: Well, I was thinking about ending therapy.

Therapist: Hmm. That's a different stance for you. I haven't ever heard you even suggest that possibility. I'm wondering what brought that up now?

Bret: Like I said, when you were away on vacation I had those extra two hours a week that we would normally be meeting, and it felt kind of good to just be living.

Therapist: Sometimes when a therapist goes on vacation people react in all sorts of ways. One way is to reject the therapist because she "abandoned" you by going on vacation. Any chance that some of that is operating here?

Bret: I don't think so. I was just looking at all the progress I made, and I was feeling pretty good being on my own. I had the time to realize I am doing well, I am doing a lot better than I had been doing.

Therapist: That sounds good, let me hear a little more.

Bret: Well, we've been working really hard, and this has been an important part of my life. I value what you say a lot. I think I've worked hard in between sessions, listening to the tapes of our sessions, taking notes on them, keeping a journal, going to meetings, and being active in my recovery program. And I think I want to try being on my own. I know I'll always be in recovery. It just seems like it might be time to eliminate this one aspect of my recovery.

Therapist: I can see what you're saying. And you may be right. You have made a lot of progress and you are doing much better. I'm just concerned about the abruptness of all this. You've been coming twice a week for a year and a half. It seems like it might make sense to reduce down to once a week, see what that's like, and talk about terminating.

Bret: You mean I can't just end this?

Therapist: Well, you can do that if you want to. But I'm suggesting you that, after all we've been through, it's a good idea for us to meet for at least six to eight weeks. We'll look at where we've been, look at what you've learned in here from me and from yourself, and kind of summarize what therapy has meant to you. Does that make sense to you? I'm suggesting a smooth and gradual withdrawal from the therapeutic process rather than an abrupt ending.

Bret: Hmm. I guess it would be kind of weird to just all of a sudden not come here anymore. You may have a point there. But I don't know about this six to eight weeks.

Therapist: I am suggesting that time frame because we have been meeting for a significant period of time and it'll take us a while to go over what we've done together and how your life has changed. Also, that's a fairly common time frame for doing a termination process in treatment. And with all that you've gained, I'd sure like this last part to be good for you also. And by good, I mean therapeutic.

I also think it's particularly important, because you have a tendency to leave and never turn back, and you once mentioned that you wanted to work on that. Here's your chance. What do you think?

Bret: Well, it's a new idea. I'd like to think about it. Can I have till next week?

Therapist: Sure.

THE SECOND WEEK

Therapist: So, how was your week?

Bret: Good. I thought a lot about what you suggested last week. And I guess I decided to go along with your suggestion about doing termination right. If there's one thing I have learned in the last year and a half, it is that I don't know everything—and most important, that I have to stay out of the driver's seat. So I'll turn this over to you and take your advice.

Therapist: You have learned a lot. Thanks for trusting me again. Let's aim for having our last session in eight weeks, okay?

Bret: Okay. What do we do for the next eight weeks?

Therapist: We can do more of what we have been doing—looking at what's happening in your life and dealing with issues that you're not sure about or that you want to check out. And we can spend some time each week looking at the progress you've made, where you were a year and a half ago, where you've been, what you've learned about yourself, how you've changed, the progress you've made, what you've learned in here, what this has meant to you, and what you think it'll be like without coming in here each week.

Bret: That's a lot.

Therapist: It is, that's why I wanted eight weeks to do it in. We don't have to do it all today.

Bret: [We both laugh] We couldn't, even if we tried. Where should we start?

Therapist: There are no hard and fast rules of where we "should" start. What about if we start at the beginning. What first brought you in here?

Bret: What first brought me in here? I was unhappy, I had recently broken up with my girlfriend, and I wanted to get another one without having to repeat the old pattern I had in relationships of leaving whenever things got too close. I had a notion that I was doing too much cocaine and that I wanted to cut down, but I didn't think I was going to have to stop completely. That was not even in my brain as a possibility. Let's see . . . Oh yeah, I also wanted to get better with my money, although I saw no relation with being broke all the time and using cocaine. I also wanted to be able to stand up to people around me and not be so wimpy all the time. I think that's about it.

Therapist: That's a good beginning. And now?

Bret: Now?

Therapist: Where are you on those things?

Bret: In much different places. You helped me to see real fast that my cocaine use had gone totally out of control, that I had to stop completely. And somehow you got it so that was an acceptable, albeit scary idea to me. And somehow—I guess that's where my higher power comes in—I was able to stop and see that I had to give up all drugs. Just from that alone, money started to stick around a little longer. I even started a savings account that has been growing steadily. So there was a link between drugs and money [He smiles].

Therapist: I remember when that notion was unacceptable to you. You refused to see the connection until the evidence was overwhelming. I think you resisted the connections between your drug use and your other problems the most. Once we were able to break through your denial, things started falling into place.

Do you remember when you realized there was a connection between "going away" with drugs and your problems with intimacy?

Bret: Oh, yeah. That was another place my stubborn denial worked against me. I didn't want to admit the power of cocaine and how powerless I had become.

I wanted my problems with intimacy to be just that—problems with intimacy and me picking the wrong people. I didn't want it to be because cocaine made me unable to deal with reality, that it was distorting my perceptions so that intimacy made me lose myself and was too frightening to maintain.

And now look at me. I followed your advice and spent the year, my first year in recovery, by myself. And like you said, I learned to like me and have fun with me. And now I've been dating this woman for, what is it? Three months now. And we get to talk about how we feel and what's going well, and what's not going so well. And I don't have to run away so much.

Therapist: You have come a long way! Are you proud of yourself? And what about gratitude?

Bret: I sure am. I remember when you first talked about pride. And the difference between false pride and real pride . . . it was scary to me because I didn't have anything to be truly proud of, and I could only voice false pride in drug bravado, and you wouldn't let me do that. I considered quitting then.

Therapist: But you didn't. And that was progress for you. You stuck with it and now you have a lot to be truly proud of and grateful for. You are now able to express and verbalize sincere feelings and reactions to all kinds of things. That's a lot of progress for you too.

Bret: It sure is. It feels good to be able to feel good. I never used to be able to do that. I am grateful that I can feel that way now.

Therapist: And how wonderful that you let yourself feel that way today. Some people can't give up the old crap, and so they stay stuck. Once things get pointed out to you, you let yourself see and take some actions on what you see. You're lucky you can do that relatively quickly. It's part of what allowed you to grow and change so much in the last year and a half.

Bret: You helped a lot too.

Therapist: Thank you. It was good to be able to be here for you. But believe me, I couldn't have done anything without your help, cooperation, and belief in recovery. You were able to get out of the driver's seat, follow advice, and try new things. That worked, and you let it work for you.

Bret: Yeah, I guess I did. It was hard at first to get out of the driver's seat and not try and control everything. But once I did, other things started falling into place real well. I still have to remember about the driver's seat, because sometimes I inadvertently wind up back in there. And then I have to pry myself out again, and remember about my higher power. Control is such an important issue in all this.

Therapist: What do you mean?

Bret: I came in here wanting to see how I could get better control over my life. I had to learn instead, how to give up control and stop trying to manipulate everybody and everything in my life. When I gave up being the director of the show, I could often respond to the little bit parts that were left just for me, and if I needed help I had places to turn.

Therapist: Look at that change. I remember you used to say how you always felt so alone, like no one was ever there for you; but instead you learned that people will be there for you if you let them, and you could let them after you stopped trying to make them do what you wanted them to do, when you wanted them to, and how you wanted them to. Then they could fall into more natural places in your life, and lo and behold, they did. You learned you don't have to be a full-time director.

Bret: That's true. I don't feel so alone anymore, and that feels good.

Therapist: We're running out of time for today. Let's meet again next week and continue this.

Bret: Okay. You know, I'm glad we decided to terminate this way. I think it would have been very hard to all of a sudden just stop coming in here.

Therapist: I'm glad you feel that way. I was hoping you would see the value in participating in a termination process.

Bret: I do. Have a good week. I'll see you next week.

Therapist: You too.

THE THIRD WEEK

Bret: What a week it's been.

Therapist: Why is that?

Bret: Well, my girlfriend went out of town for a long weekend to see her parents and I missed her. I really did. I missed her so much that I seriously contemplated breaking up with her. You know that I'm not allowed to feel too close. Luckily, when I went to a meeting someone was talking about a similar set of circumstances and I realized, that breaking up or wanting to, was my crazy thinking, and I had to let go and get past that craziness. I struggled with that for a few days. But I shared with her what was happening, so when I was a little erratic she was pretty understanding. She didn't overwhelm me with her needs and accepted that I was struggling, which probably made it easier for me not to give in to the old craziness and I got past it. I know I like her a lot, enough to miss her, and I'm entitled to that— even if an old sick part of me doesn't think so.

Therapist: It sounds like you really worked that one out. Congratulations. You must feel good about that.

Bret: I do. I really do, but I was wondering if I'm terminating too quickly. When something like that happens I get scared and wonder if I'm being premature. You know, there are still things I want to work on and change.

Therapist: I hope there'll always be things you'll want to work on and change. That's part of being alive and vital and human. As for whether you're being premature or not, I can't be sure. It doesn't seem like you are. Here was a good test, in a sense, for you. And yes, you struggled for a few days, and your old craziness came back, but your new ways of coping with life were effective. Even if you stayed in therapy for twenty years you would not be eliminating struggles like this one. We're human and we'll never be perfect. The trick is to have people and resources (like your higher power) you can rely on for support. It sounds like you handled a tough week very well.

Do you have some other reasons why all of a sudden ending therapy doesn't seem like such a great idea?

Bret: Nothing very concrete, except this week, when I thought of what ending really meant—not coming in here and seeing you, talking things out with you— I was upset and scared. Upset because I've come to value what you say. And I'll miss hearing your input and having your caring. It's been very important to me. Your opinions, all your input, have at times been such necessary reality checks when I've been so sub-jectively distorted in my view of reality. I don't really want to lose that in my life.

Therapist: That's very nice to hear. It's touching. It truly is. You said you didn't want to lose my perspective, my input—you won't ever lose it. After this long you've incorporated some of it—that which makes most sense to you—into your own way of thinking. You'll take what you've learned from me and in these ses-sions always, wherever you go. That's one of the presents of a good therapeutic process. You get extras that you always have, inside you.

Bret: Hmm.

Therapist: You can also come back if you really feel the need, either for short-term or long-term work. And my caring, that'll always be there. Even if you don't get a direct hit of it each week, you can be sure that I'm out here rooting for you.

Bret: Oh, yeah?

Therapist: What do you think? That after working with you this intensely for a year and a half I would just, upon termination, close you out, never again to think about you? Of course I wonder and hope for the best for you. Please don't forget that learning in here is a two-way street. I have learned from you, too. You've made an impact on my life. If I'm not learning in here, good work isn't happening.

Bret: Oh, come on, I was such a mess when I came in here. What could you have possibly learned from me?

Therapist: Is that a self-deprecating note I hear?

Bret: [Laughing] Probably not a note; it's more like a chorus.

Therapist: Would you like to ask that question a little differently?

Bret: That sounds like a good idea. What have you learned from me?

Therapist: A lot. I'll have to think about that for a while to give you a complete answer. But one of the things I learned was how much courage it took you to face things in your life, and how you managed to find that courage even as you insisted there was none there. Remember when you were acting like such a wimp? Not standing up for yourself, allowing people to walk all over you? Working in a job you hated but were too "afraid to quit?" Remember back then?

Bret: [Smiling] I sure do. Ugh! And I never want to revisit the land of the living wimps. That's how I view that part of my life, I had temporarily dropped into the land of the living wimps, kind of how Dorothy landed in the Land of Oz.

Therapist: Well, you found the courage to leave. And I learned a lot about people's hidden talents and abilities when you began to emerge from what you call the land of the living wimps . . .

Bret: You learned from that?

Therapist: Yes, I did.

Bret: But I was being such a jerk.

Therapist: That's how you see it. I saw someone who was so stuck by so many nameless fears that I wasn't sure you could ever get out. And I certainly didn't think it would take such a short amount of time. But once you made that first breakthrough you were on your way. There was no stopping you.

Bret: There were some backslides along the way.

Therapist: So?

Bret: Well, I wasn't perfect?

Therapist: Is that what you're aiming for? Because if you are, you're in for a big surprise, and a bigger disappointment. Remember about perfection?

Bret: What about it?

Therapist: One minor detail . . . it doesn't exist.

Bret: Oh, I know that.

Therapist: I know you know that, but you either temporarily just forgot that you knew it or you were fishing for a compliment or looking for a way to put yourself down. You still do that. Maybe that's one of the things you can continue to work on and try to let go of. Maybe you could even turn it over to your higher power.

Bret: My putting myself down?

Therapist: That's what I was suggesting.

Bret: You're probably right. This week, for instance, I had trouble seeing past the fact that it was a tough week, to how much differently I handled it, and how pleased I could be at how differently I did handle it.

Therapist: Do you see it now?

Bret: Yes, I do.

Therapist: Good, be grateful for that, because there was a time when you might not have seen it so quickly.

Bret: That's true. I sure have learned a lot.

Therapist: You sure have. It's getting late. See you next week?

Bret: I'll be here.

THE FOURTH WEEK

Bret: I had a much better week this week than the week
            before.

Therapist: What do you attribute that to?

Bret: I let it happen.

Therapist: You let it happen?

Bret: I didn't fight feeling good. And I acknowledged my-
            self instead of finding fault all the time.

Therapist: And how did that feel?

Bret: Real good!

Therapist: Well, that's great.

Bret: Thanks.

Therapist: You're very welcome.

Bret: I feel a little better about terminating, too.

Therapist: Good. What's that about?

Bret: I listened to what you said last week about always
            having some of you and what I've learned in here
            with me. And I think it's true. I also know that I
            don't want to be in therapy forever, and I have made
            a lot of progress . . . I just get a little sad when I
            think about not having your support every week.

Therapist: I think that's a natural response. There is going to
            be a loss when you no longer have this therapeutic
            relationship in your life. But not all losses are nega-
            tive. You'll be moving on to something very exciting
            and challenging and rewarding—life. And you have
            some supports that will always be there—meetings,
            a higher power, and lots of other people in recovery.

So it's okay to feel sad. It probably means this meant a lot to you.

Bret: It has. I'm surprised I didn't realize how much it has meant till now.

Therapist: Lots of times when we're involved in something we start forgetting to notice things about it that make it special to us. That can happen in all kinds of relationships—work, friends, and therapeutic relationships. Who was it who said, "You have to stop and smell the flowers along the way"? Right now you're taking the time to smell the therapeutic flowers you've planted along the way. I hope you'll keep allowing yourself to do just that and enjoy the details of what you've created.

Bret: But I don't like to feel sad.

Therapist: Why not?

Bret: It hurts.

Therapist: It hurts? Does it just hurt? What about crying?

Bret: It does hurt, the loss part hurts. But I can see what you mean, the tears can be a relief and a release. And with endings come beginnings, but I'm always afraid of beginnings.

Therapist: A certain amount of fear or trepidation or anticipation at beginnings is appropriate. You don't know what's beyond . . . just as long as you don't let your fears paralyze you. And you haven't let them do that in a long time. You know how to get help and let go of your fears.

Bret: That's true, I do. Something else you just said about fear or trepidation or anticipation being okay to have . . . You know, I might do well to rename a few feelings and not always call them fears. There is a range of emotions, like you just suggested, that are good to have that might keep me on my toes rather than being overwhelmed and feeling helpless and wimpish.

Therapist: What other emotions might you have that would feel appropriate at times?

Bret: Excitement, looking forward to something. You know, I used to think there was fear, good, and bad. That was it. All emotions had to fit into one of those three categories. And then I started experiencing "okay"—I mean just feeling okay, not quite good and not quite bad. It was awkward at first, because I couldn't pigeonhole that feeling, although I sure did try. And then I felt what I came to learn was pride one day. When I stayed clean for one whole week and felt a slight swelling in my chest, after I ruled out a heart attack I realized I was feeling some pride in myself. From there the floodgates of emotions have opened up quite a bit for me.

Feeling sad was always a bad feeling, and now you're suggesting that there can be some joy with sadness, and that's new for me to think about. But I understand what you mean. There's another feeling, understanding. You know, you have to let go of some self-consciousness to truly feel understanding with another human being. Understanding, sympathy, and empathy—those are all feelings that were quite foreign to me a year and a half ago. But they're more common these days. I even like them. It's fun to be able to relate to people.

My wall of fears and my self-consciousness that backed up those fears had prevented me from knowing people for so long. It's a shame that I was so handicapped by that wall. I'm glad I got past it.

See, in the past I would now start obsessing about what a shame it is that I had been so handicapped by the wall. Instead I want to celebrate getting past the wall.

Therapist: You certainly deserve to do just that.

Bret: I know I do. And knowing that is different, and progress also.

Therapist: You're right.

Bret: I realized this week that I was trying, a few times, to do what you often do in here.

Therapist: What's that?

Bret: I was trying to stand back and assess what I was doing or saying and take it more in a positive way— you know, be reinforcing like you are. I guess I've been being nicer to myself. I figure since you won't be in my life in a few weeks, if I like that happening I better do it for myself. I thought of that and started doing it after going over what you had said about learning from you and always having that as a gift with me at all times. I like that, but I thought I'd better practice at it before I left therapy, so I would get better at it and could iron out any kinks before we terminated.

Therapist: [Smiling] Good idea.

Bret: Thanks.

Therapist: How's the rest of your life treating you?

Bret: Good. I'm enjoying work again. The people are not bothering me as much. I've let myself off the hook; when they complain, I no longer feel like it's all my fault or that I have to figure out how to make them feel better. I do my job, listen to them, and sometimes I can understand their feelings and sympathize with them, but I'm no longer the culprit.

It was pretty crazy how I had gotten myself into that role. Pretty crazy and pretty grandiose to think I was to blame for all their troubles. I laugh sometimes when I think back to how I used to feel. Somehow even when they were having personal troubles I construed it to mean that if I was a better manager they would be happier at work and therefore happier and not fighting with their spouses or partners . . . That's pretty crazy.

Therapist: I won't argue with you on that one. I'm glad you've got that in perspective now.

Bret: Me too. All that crap was a heavy burden to be carrying around all the time.

Therapist: I bet it was. How are you doing with other aspects of your recovery?

Bret: Good. I still get so much out of meetings I go to. Rarely do I go to one where nobody says anything I can relate to. It's much more the case that I can relate to what people are saying and learn from it. I still have trouble speaking in the larger meetings, although I do push myself. I like the smaller meetings and speak up frequently in them. I like sharing. I'll probably do that more when I don't have your undivided attention anymore. I may go to more meetings. Now I go to two or three a week, depending on how I feel. I like being flexible about the number; it makes me feel like this is more something I want to be doing than something I have to be doing.

Therapist: That sounds good. Actually, all of what you're saying today sounds good and healthy. How are you feeling about terminating at this point? We have four more sessions, but how is that feeling?

Bret: Better again. I know I initiated this . . . I have my doubts—but I feel better knowing I can come back if I want to.

Therapist: You can come back. One of the reasons I feel good about you terminating now is that you have learned a lot; you're getting better and better at being nice to yourself and letting things go. In therapy, like in all other areas of your life, you have to be careful not to get too dependent. I don't want you to need me in your life for you to live a relatively happy and healthy life. That doesn't work. You need to be able to give yourself and get happiness and health outside a therapeutic setting and without paying for it. It feels like you are going to be able to do just that, and I'm glad you can. So, for me, it does feel more and more like our timing on this termination process is right.

Bret: Me too.

Therapist: This session went quickly.

Bret: It's time already? I'll see you next week.

THE FIFTH WEEK

Therapist: How are you doing?

Bret: Good. I'm still enjoying myself.

Therapist: Is that a little surprise I hear in your voice?

Bret: [Laughing] Yes, you know me, I'm still not quite used to feeling good. That impending feeling of doom isn't quite right over my shoulder breathing cold shudders of air down my back. It's at least a few steps in back of me. I can still see it from the periphery of my vision at times, but I just tell it to go away. And now it listens a lot of the time. Can you imagine that?

Therapist: [Laughing] I think so. What happens when it doesn't listen?

Bret: You had to bring that up, didn't you? No, really, I'm joking. When it doesn't listen sometimes I tell it, "Then fine, stick around and have some fun if you want." Other times I get caught by it and I feel scared for a while. But I don't get lost in it like I used to. I can let it go, or when it hangs around for more than a few hours or maybe for more than a day, I call someone and talk about it or I go to a meeting. AA meetings have a marvelous knack of getting rid of the doom. It's almost like it gets checked and thrown away as I enter the room.

If it still insists on meeting me later on the outside, I try to just let it linger, and I don't get freaked out by it. I assume it gets bored and leaves because I just realize it's not there anymore. I figure my doom may stick around for a while. I just hope I can stay out of its firm grip; so far I seem to be.

And then, like you've said, that's a feeling too. So when all else fails, I try to remind myself of the image you presented of feelings like waves coming and going—then I know that this, too, will pass.

Therapist: I'm impressed with how well you are doing and all the differences we've been talking about in the last few weeks. Do you realize what a long way you've come?

Bret: I'm beginning to. This termination process is very helpful in bringing all that out. I'm trying to dwell on what I've learned in here and incorporate all that into my life more, instead of leaving it all up to you and depending on an hour or two a week to get my reinforcement. I'm pleased that I can do this kind of thing so well during the week. I hadn't realized I had learned so much.

Therapist: How are you dealing with other people?

Bret: Around this type of thing?

Therapist: Yes.

Bret: Funny you should ask that.

Therapist: Funny?

Bret: My girlfriend and I were talking about just that subject last night. She was saying that she was seeing a big change in me.

Therapist: What is she seeing?

Bret: She said that I seem to be easier on myself lately, and as I'm easier on myself I seem more accepting of her. She said it wasn't even necessarily on a verbal level, I just seemed to have relaxed some more or let up some more in the last few weeks. She hopes it lasts.

Therapist: And you?

Bret: I hope it lasts too.

Therapist: What are some differences in how you're feeling?

Bret: You know, this may sound kind of crazy, but I feel lighter, as if I've shed about twenty pounds.

Therapist: I believe that. You look more relaxed in here. Even the way you sit—you aren't quite gripping the arms of the chair the way you used to.

Bret: I think I know what you mean. It was almost like I was holding on against the onslaught I thought would be coming. That had to do with that impending sense of doom I walked around with. I felt like I had to brace against "It"—but I'm not sure what "it" was.

Therapist: Maybe the twenty-pound weight drop is letting go of your armor.

Bret: Like that heavy metal stuff the knights used to wear?

Therapist: That was my image.

Bret: It sure fits.

Therapist: It also sounds like you're letting your girlfriend in a little closer.

Bret: Yes, that is happening, too.

Therapist: You said that as if you weren't doing anything, and somehow she got closer.

Bret: It seems that way, although I didn't realize that was how I was saying it. You're right. I'm just not fighting it and it's happening. I'm not sure if she's "the one," and I don't have to know that right now. But it sure feels good, and we are having a good time. So I, for one, am not fighting a good thing.

Therapist: That's nice to hear . . .

Bret: I agree. I want to thank you for all your patience and help. I know I haven't been the most cooperative person to work with at times, and I sure am glad you've hung in there with me. I couldn't have gotten here without you. I'll never forget what has happened in this room. It's been like magic sometimes, how I can hear things you say in here that I'm sure other people must have said to me at various times, but I couldn't hear it before.

Therapist: It's been a pleasure watching you grow and blossom. As for the occasional uncooperativeness, that's part of the business, to be expected. I wouldn't want someone to just take everything I said at face value and not question it at least some of the time. Otherwise you would get too dependent on me and not learn how to think for yourself. And if everything I said turned out to be words of wisdom, my ego would get too inflated. And then we'd all be in trouble. [Laughing] Your "uncooperativeness" is part of the therapeutic process and part of your exploring, questioning, and growing. It has been necessary—yes, sometimes a pain in the neck—but a necessary pain in the neck. [Smiling]

I'm not sure I agree with you when you say you couldn't have gotten here without me. There are lots of roads that bring you to the same place, the ride might have been different, but you got here and that's what's important. I have been glad to help when I could, and, as I say, it has been a pleasure for me to see you give up drugs and learn to live and be a lot happier without them. That, in and of itself, has been very rewarding for me.

Bret: I like what you just said. Well, we have three more weeks together, right?

Therapist: That's it. How do you feel knowing that?

Bret: I'm beginning to feel nostalgic already. You've been real important to me and I'll miss you. I'm glad I've been able to develop friendships outside of here so I have a number of people in my daily life who are real important to me also. That's not to take away from what happens in here; it's just the first time I've had such a solid support group in my life; it feels very healthy. So it won't be like I'll have nothing when we stop seeing each other and therapy is over in three more weeks.

Therapist: I know that. I don't think I would have let you terminate as easily if I was the only support in your life. If you weren't yet able to form healthy, supportive relationships and friendships, it would have indicated that you were not ready to terminate. The fact that you have friends now, in the true sense of the word, is all the more indicative of your progress and your readiness for terminating.

Bret: You really think so?

Therapist: Don't you?

Bret: Yeah. I hadn't thought of it like that, but I agree.

Therapist: Time has passed quickly again. Good session. See you next week.

Bret: Okay.

THE SIXTH WEEK

Bret: Well, I'm doing okay, but I'm worrying a lot about my job. It seems like it's been on my mind a lot this week.

Therapist: Been on your mind in a good sense or an overly obsessive way?

Bret: Bordering on both and ricocheting back and forth between the two.

Therapist: Tell me some more.

Bret: Well, you know I haven't been very happy with my work for a long time. I don't feel like I get enough freedom for my creativity in my job. I'm a good interior designer, but everything I do is checked and double checked by my manager and his manager.

And they never give good feedback. I have to figure out how well I've done by the number of negative comments I get, and the less I get the better I did. I'm tired of that. I want to be treated better. I'm beginning to wonder if it's time to start branching out on my own or finding a job with another firm.

Therapist: You know, I believe that this is happening right now for you on a very real level. But I have to point out to you that often, at this point in the termination process, people tend to come up with a crisis of big enough proportion to justify staying in therapy. For the last five weeks you've been going over your progress to date; you've been enjoying feeling good for a prolonged time; how much of this is hidden "I don't really want to terminate"?

Bret: That's quite a mouthful. It's kind of hard to hear. Yes, I think this is real. My feelings of dissatisfaction on the job have been mounting for months, and you know that. So I know that is real. Whether the panic-like state I've been bordering on all week has to be the response, I don't know, and frankly I wish it wasn't there, but it is. It felt good to know I could come in here and you would probably be able to help.

Therapist: I think I can help best by asking you what you want to do about your job and how you want to be able to handle these escalating feelings of dissatisfaction on the job.

Bret: You're putting it back on me?

Therapist: Yes. I want you to know you can do this. We have two more sessions after today, and I want you to prove to yourself that you can handle this.

Bret: Then why am I paying you?

Therapist:	That feels like some anger coming at me. What's that about?
Bret:	I thought you were supposed to do that?
Therapist:	Come up with solutions?
Bret:	Yeah!
Therapist:	I haven't done that in a long time. I've been guiding you more to come up with your own.
Bret:	But I want you to do it. You know my situation.
Therapist:	I'm wondering why you want me to do it instead of you? Where's this new-found dependence coming from?
Bret:	Wait a minute, I thought you were supposed to be supportive? Now you sound like my boss.
Therapist:	If I really do, maybe you need to reassess how you are hearing what he's saying.
	You know, I don't think we're talking about your job situation at all. It feels like that's a cover-up for some termination feelings you have, but that it's not okay for some reason for you to express them directly. Do you know what I mean?
Bret:	I think so. It's just that I was feeling so good about terminating. Why is all this happening now? I wanted it to be smooth, and now I'm messing it up. I can't do anything right.
Therapist:	Hold on there a minute. First of all, you said you wanted it to be smooth. That's a nice wish, but since when can you control everything? Aren't all feelings valid when they're in response to a real situation? Since when was terminating a process that only involved good feelings? I told you we would have to deal with loss and sadness and probably some grief.

It seems like you're dealing with them by masking them as anger instead. And by thinking of leaving another fairly set routine in your life as well. Maybe one thing at a time? But if it's time to move on in your job, handle that too—only try to keep it separate from this. And right now it's pretty muddy . . .

Do you really believe yourself when you say, "I can't do anything right"?

Bret: [With a chagrin] No. Not really. You know I was just feeling sorry for myself.

Therapist: Well, I didn't know that for sure. I'm glad you've clarified that. What about the rest of what I said?

Bret: You're probably pretty accurate in what you're saying. My anger is probably sadness, and it's easier for me to leave angry; then I don't turn back as much as I'm walking away. So, I was probably trying to get you so angry you'd tell me to leave now, or me so angry I wouldn't want to come back; then I could terminate with no regrets.

Therapist: And in the process you get to make shit out of something really good.

Bret: Yeah, I do. But that's how I've always done it.

Therapist: I know, we've talked about it. And, if at all possible, you said you don't want to do it again. Do you want to try a different way of doing it?

Bret: Yes. I do. Thanks for stopping me.

Therapist: Thanks for listening. You didn't have to stop as easily as you did. You were really ready.

Bret: You think so?

Therapist: Yes. Now are you ready to try something different?

Bret: I just said I was. What are we going to do?

Therapist: Not "we," *you*. You are going to sit back, take a couple of deep breaths, and when you are ready tell me about your feelings of loss and sadness that seep in when you think about not coming in here anymore. And if you can't think of any on your own, ask for some help from your higher power.

Bret: That's a hard one.

Therapist: I never said this was easy. Are you willing?

Bret: Okay. I'm sitting back.

Therapist: Now just relax, take a couple of deep breaths, and let your feelings come to the surface; when you're ready you can talk about them.

Bret: . . . I get this image that I'm lost at sea. Not exactly lost, but that I'm adrift. I can see some lighthouses off in the distance, not even so far away, but I'm not sure I can get there. I guess I know I can, but I'm not sure it's worth the effort.

Therapist: What does that mean to you?

Bret: I know I have other people I can reach out to, but I'm not sure they'll really be there for me.

Therapist: How does that tie in with leaving here?

Bret: I've always known you would be here for me. I've never had a person in my life who I was sure would be there for me like you've been.

Therapist: And?

Bret: And I'm not so sure I'm ready to lose that, and I'm not so sure my support system I've created is going to be as dependable as you.

Therapist: And if they're not?

Bret: I'm not sure what you're asking me.

Therapist: If they are not as dependable as I've been?

Bret: Oh, I don't know.

Therapist: Can you look for more that would be more dependable?

Bret: I suppose.

Therapist: And aren't you a lot more dependable than you've ever been?

Bret: Me?

Therapist: You. You're your own best friend. You need to be the most dependable. How are you feeling about your support system?

Bret: If I stand back, I know in my head it is fine. But my quakey guts wonder if this is too good to be real.

Therapist: What can you do about your quakey guts?

Bret: Test them?

Therapist: Are you asking me?

Bret: Well, I'm offering that as one possibility.

Therapist: Are there others?

Bret: Trust them and prove to myself by reaching out that people will be there.

Therapist: That's right. And please know that at times people won't be able to be there and respond as you would like them to, because they'll be caught in their own stuff, and that's okay. You'll still have yourself, your higher power, and your recovery program.

Bret: I have to remember that.

Therapist: Usually, you do.

Bret: But I have to always remember that.

Therapist: Always? Remember, nothing's perfect.

Bret: Oh, yeah. I better remember that, too. Oh, look at that. It's time again. This was a heavy session.

Therapist: And we dealt with some things we have to deal with. Let yourself spend some time this week feeling sad and feeling the loss if you need to.

Bret: I will.

THE SEVENTH WEEK

Therapist: So, how was your week?

Bret: A mixed bag. I spent a good deal of time depressed, and some time feeling good that I was letting myself be depressed and sad.

Therapist: Sounds like you stopped running away from your feelings and that you lifted your ban on negative feelings other than anger.

Bret: That's a funny way of putting it . . . My girlfriend said it was pretty hard being around me this week. I tried to share with her how I was feeling, but I guess I wasn't doing enough of that. She said I got better as the week went on.

Therapist: What did you think?

Bret: What did I think about what?

Therapist: You just said she said it got better as the week went on. How did you feel about yourself and how you were interacting with her?

Bret: If I face the truth, I think I did do better. At first I think I was trying to shut her out with my sadness and depression. And then later I think I was letting her know more about what I was going through. I think on a crazy level, when I couldn't get you to reject me with my anger last week, I tried to get her to reject me through my depression and going away that way. Then when that didn't work, I realized what I was doing and I decided to try something different.

Therapist: So you were able to catch yourself and switch how you were acting to something that was more functional for you.

Bret: Yeah.

Therapist: You broke a bad pattern instead of wallowing in it.

Bret: I guess that is what I did.

Therapist: What's with your job?

Bret: I'm still fairly dissatisfied, but I think I'll wait a while to make a move. I know, realistically, that if I'm going to try and open my own business I have to have a lot of money backing me up, which I don't have but am saving towards. So I have to decide if I want to switch to another firm, or stay put where at least I know what to expect.

Therapist: How does that feel?

Bret: It feels like the most rational thing to be doing. I think you had some insights that I agree with last week about why I was looking to leave right now. And it's not that intolerable. I can stay for a while. I want to leave for something better if I leave, and not just make a brash decision. I know how hard it is to find a job in this city. And a great way to sabotage myself would be to quit without another job lined up, and then go through all my savings so my dream of having my own business would be farther away. Or I could even look at it as lost for now, and then I could get really upset and go into quite a tailspin.

Therapist: It sounds like you have that scenario worked out already.

Bret: It's the scenario I know would have been on automatic in the old days, and one I would like to avert if at all possible.

Therapist: It sounds like you have a head start on averting it.

Bret: I hope so. You know, you suggested I spend some time feeling those difficult feelings of sadness and loss and grief—well, I did, and what I came up with was that I want to find people in my life who will be as healthy for me as you have been. I've learned from you that people can be trusted and they can help each other. I know that once in a while people in my life have tried to teach me or be like that before, but I couldn't see it. And now I can. I realized how much I like people who care and reach out to others, and I'm going to continue to look for people like that in my life.

One way I can do that is to stand up for what I want and believe in and not take shit that people dish out. I want to keep the old wimp in me retired. If I can do that, then the loss from losing this therapeutic relationship won't be as startling and as long lasting, because the loss is going to be far outweighed by the gains I have. And like you said weeks ago, nobody can take those away.

Therapist: Do you also remember that it was you who initiated this termination process? I wasn't so sure when you first brought it up. It seemed so abrupt, but as you talked on I had to respect what you said and agree with your reasons. Nobody is taking anything away from you; you chose to move on.

Bret: You know, I had forgotten that.

Therapist: It was beginning to sound like you had.

Bret: So, next week is our last session.

Therapist: Yes, it is.

Bret: Do you want me to think about anything special?

Therapist: Just what you'd like to get out of the last session.

Bret: That sounds easy enough. See you next week.

THE EIGHTH AND FINAL WEEK

Bret: Well, this is it.

Therapist: It sure is. What did you think about and come up with this week?

Bret: I was thinking of looking back on our very first session, and I was curious to hear what you thought of me that first week and how you've seen me change since then.

Therapist: Okay, I'll do that if you'll do the same after me. That way we get both perspectives.

Bret: It's a deal.

Therapist: Let's see. The first session. First of all, you were a physical mess. I could tell you had gone to some lengths to look presentable, because your shirt was badly ironed and your pants had been hemmed, although the tape from your hemming job was falling down. You were very skinny; it looked like you hadn't been eating well by your extreme thinness and pallid color of your cheeks.

Bret: You remember all that?

Therapist: Well, I've been thinking about this too. Let's see. You were very fidgety, especially after you whipped out a cigarette and I told you this was a no-smoking office. You didn't like that at all. In fact, you mentioned that you might have to leave and take a cigarette break. If I recall correctly, I said you were welcome to do that, but we had fifty minutes together and that's what you were paying me for. So if you took a break it would still be considered part of the session. You didn't take that cigarette break and never again mentioned a need for one. I saw that as a hopeful sign.

You also came in here wanting to cut back on your cocaine use, but when I talked to you about cocaine use, abuse, and addiction, and what had to follow if you were addicted, you were surprisingly cooperative—at first . . . You did argue later on, but only after you had slipped a few times and were not sure you wanted to have to give up all drugs and come in here and go to meetings. That seemed too much for you. But that battle only lasted a few weeks and then you decided to try recovery with the attitude of "what did I have to lose?" And from that point on you started gaining, not losing.

You started gaining weight, doing better on your job, looking at feelings you had kept down with drugs for a long time. Sure, once in a while things were hard for you to accept, but you kept coming back. And that's the key. You wanted to learn how to deal with your disease. You were willing. And it worked for you. You started making some friends, even going outside and getting some color. I remember when you played tennis for the first time in seven years and you came in and said you were bad, but at least you were on the tennis court again.

It seems like one of the biggest changes for you is, as you say, retiring your wimpish mask and beginning to stand up as a person and be able to reach out to others, getting support and giving support. I tell you, I was pretty sure you could get here. I just wasn't at all sure how long it would take you. It seemed like it would take you a lot longer, but you made it. You people who like cocaine tend to be fast movers. [Smiling]

Bret: [Laughing] That is true, isn't it? I've noticed that a lot of cocaine addicts at meetings have a lot of energy. That's probably part of what attracted us to the drug so much, that extra energy boost we got from it. It was great at first, till it turned on us. But I tell you, this natural energy I get is so much better than what I used to get when I was using. I'm so thankful I found this way of being, because I was sure looking intensely for it with drugs and not finding it in a hurry. Meanwhile, I was racing downstream all along and didn't even know it.

I remember our first session, but it's a little more hazy than you recall. I had gone on a hefty run the weekend before coming in here, so I was pretty wired and out of it when I came in. My impressions, as I remember them, were that you were talking a lot of shit that I didn't want to hear about addiction and what the cocaine was doing to me; but even as I didn't want to hear it, something inside me knew you were right. That's why I came back the next week. Because I knew you were making sense.

And for about the first month that's what kept me coming back. I knew you knew what you were talking about, and even if I didn't want to hear it I knew I had to hear it. Then I remember the session where you said it was okay if I didn't believe what you said wholeheartedly, but that I could just act as if I did believe it and see what happened. That was a real turning point for me.

I started going to meetings more frequently, coming in here and listening more openly. And "acting as if" lasted a while, till I realized that I truly wanted what recovery had to offer: a saner, more spiritual life, where I didn't have to be in the driver's seat all the time. And life became so much more bearable. It was all such a relief for me. It's real clear that when I was trying to manage everything and everybody I was making quite a mess of myself. Not having to take care of it all was quite a relief and worked much better.

I guess things started mushrooming from there. I met some people at meetings and became friends with some of them. I even met some new people and started developing friendships with people through my work associations. And I started seeing what being alive is like, I even started enjoying it. It just seems like that kept continuing, and I kept peeling off layers of an onion called me, shedding what didn't work anymore and keeping what did. I still have some layers I'd rather not have—but, like you say, nobody's perfect. At least, I know better how to deal with those bothersome layers.

Therapist: You sure have come a long way.

Bret: I sure have.

Therapist: I want to thank you for all your acknowledgment of my help. That feels nice. I couldn't have done it without your active participation in a full recovery program.

You've learned well how to deal with your disease; you know what it takes to stay clean. I hope you keep allowing yourself to do what it takes.

Bret: Me too. I'm also glad I have the option of coming back here if I really need to. Don't worry—I won't run back at the first crisis that comes along. I don't want to get dependent on you either. It's just good to know you'd be interested.

Therapist: You bet. And don't be surprised to hear from me every now and again. I will make follow-up phone calls to see how you're doing. And you can call me every once in a while, too, to catch me up if you'd like.

Bret: Good, I may do that. Thank you so much for everything.

Therapist: And thank you. Take care.

Bret: I will, and you too.

Therapist: I intend to.

Bret: Well, I guess that's it.

Therapist: I guess so.

Bret: This is a little weird. All I have to do is leave, but . . .

Therapist: Come on, I'll walk you to the door.

Bret: That's better.

Therapist: Want a hug?

Bret: You bet. [Client and therapist hug. Client looks around the office] Boy, a lot has happened in here.

Therapist: You did. Now keep doing what you learned, and you'll do fine.

Bret: I hope to do just that.

Termination can be a very positive experience for both client and therapist. It is a leave taking process that therapeutically can establish new ways of making endings and moving on to new things. During the six- to eight-week process, the client is usually able to experience a range of feelings from pride to humbleness, from sadness to joy, from depression to anger, and all points in between.

I see the termination process as a microcosm of the entire therapeutic relationship. Usually, all feelings are reexperienced as both people look at where they've been together and what they've learned from each other. Last-minute transferential issues are dealt with again, and laid to rest. It is a final growth experience for the client with the therapist as progress is reviewed and goals are set. Termination marks the beginning of an individual recovery process that will, ideally, last the person's whole lifetime.

Epilogue: A New Beginning

Throughout this book I have tried to present stories that reflect the lives, problems, and struggles that the people I have worked with have actually experienced. These stories are not meant as a scare tactic; rather, they have been reflections of reality, a reality that is not often discussed among cocaine users, abusers, or addicts. But it should be.

Perhaps this book can spark some new discussions about all angles of the cocaine reality. It has been written as a beginning to a much-needed educational campaign on the realities of cocaine use, abuse, and addiction. The realities are not just for the user, but for family, friends, and work associates who are affected by the user's behavior. Cocaine is indeed the most insidious drug we know—insidious because it is so seductive, so alluring, so mystical, and ultimately so addictive and destructive.

At this moment, even as you read this, millions of American people are using cocaine. They may be snorting a few lines right now in their corporate office bathrooms. They may be at a party freebasing, or in a room shooting some into their veins. Many will check for telltale signs: cleaning white powder from their nostrils, rolling down their sleeves to hide their tracks, hiding the freebase pipe so they won't be found out. Others will not even care; they are either too cocky or too oblivious. All these cocaine users have one thing in common: they believe they are having fun. Incredibly, millions of otherwise intelligent people are happily entering a trap door labeled "cocaine" that will alter their lives forever.

National statistics claim that two out of every ten people who use cocaine recreationally will become addicted. All cocaine users assume they are part of that safe eight. None see themselves as potential addicts. Yet, because cocaine is an illegal drug (which precludes accurate figures) and denial of addiction is so strong, one even wonders if the two in ten approximation is correct. After working with cocaine addicts for the last few years, I think the ratio is higher. Perhaps my sample is biased by the nature of my clients and the fact that I live and work in San Francisco.

If I do not have a biased sample and my clients and my social experiences during the last few years are representative of a nationwide trend (which it seems to be), then I think this country is in trouble—in trouble because a lot of people are walking around addicted and not knowing or admitting they have a problem, and therefore not getting any help. Hence a lot of other people at home and at work are being affected by distorted perceptions, thoughts, and emotions. The problem of cocaine addiction is widespread—by national statistics we are talking about millions of people (and, if you add in cocaine abuse, the reality can be staggering); the consequences on the functioning of this country could be far-reaching.

At this year's Ninth Annual Comedy Competition in San Francisco, I was struck by how many jokes involved cocaine. It is a popular social subject. I overhear many innuendos in social and professional circles, all pertaining to that popular white powder, cocaine. I wonder why it is so popular, why people think they have to be high or loaded in order to have a good time. Recently, a client of mine who has been clean for about six months came in and was very agitated; she started the session by saying:

Joanne, I'm just beginning to feel what it's like to be clearheaded all the time and I like it. But what has me really upset is, why did I and why do all those other people out there get high all the time? I mean, what does that say? Don't they realize what they're doing? I know I didn't, but I'm an addict. What about them? Even so-called social users, they are putting something in their system that is distorting their thinking, it's clouding their mind. And they don't realize it.

Why in America is it so okay to be getting high all the time? To have a martini or two at lunch and then go back to the office and try to function? Or a few martinis at night—what's that showing the kids? I can't believe how judgmental I'm getting but I'm just beginning to see clearly and I'm really scared about what's happening in this country. Is it only in this country, or around the world? What about politicians? When's the last time there was a state dinner without wine? And they are making decisions that will affect the whole world for a long time. Joanne, I tell you, it's scary.

Many people I have worked with have had similar reactions when they begin to experience what it is like to be drug-free. They are appalled at our societal sanctions for using drugs. Alcohol is certainly the most acceptable drug; but cocaine, in certain circles, is equally acceptable. I can remember being at parties where people who refused to partake in the various drugs that were offered (wine, beer, hard liquor, and marijuana) were accused of having turned in their "hard-core badges," of not being able to "keep up" with the rest of the crowd. Peer pressure can be very powerful. It is often not as overt as asking where your hard-core badge is, but just by their very presence drugs call out for people to use them, especially a drug as seductive as cocaine.

When clients get upset as they realize how many people around them use and abuse drugs and what that means in terms of those peoples' cognitive and emotional functioning, we discuss that reality. We also discuss the need for them to focus on their own recovery and not be judge and jury for the rest of the world. They have to be careful not to start one-person crusades. But our discussions do bring up interesting questions: Why is it that so many people associate having fun with getting high or getting loaded? Having a drink or two is not enough a lot of the time; the goal is to get high, to alter your state of consciousness considerably. Why is being who they are so unacceptable to so many people? Why do so many people think they have to have drugs around to attract another person? Why do people think they have to put some mood-altering chemical into their system in order to have fun at a party or enjoy a concert or have a significant discussion? What does all this say about our society? Our values? I think it is appropriate that people get concerned about these things as they are getting clean and sober, and as they are formulating a new drug-free lifestyle that will work for them. It is a sobering topic for thought.

Writing this book has been helpful to me. It has been a way to take a step back and look at my own work. I have seen very graphically how my own therapeutic style has grown and developed over the last few years. I hope this book will be understood as having been based on what we know about cocaine and chemical dependency treatment today, an understanding that may change over time. Right now, we know the disease model is the most effective model for treatment we have to offer. Maybe someday scientists will isolate a genetic or biochemical factor that predisposes a person to addiction, but we are just not there yet. And even then we might still have addictive thinking to contend with. Right now we can work with addiction as a disease that is relapsable and chronic, but also treatable.

One of the main ingredients for any successful recovery program is abstinence from all drugs. Cocaine addicts are not exceptions to this rule. A lot of what you have read here applies to any kind of chemical dependency. You can substitute alcohol, pills, marijuana, heroin, or any other drug for cocaine, and a lot of these principles still apply. Cocaine addicts sometimes cry out for special treatment; but they are addicts and need to be treated that way. Their addiction may be psychological rather than physical in nature, but I have learned that addiction is addiction; treatment doesn't vary whether the addiction is psychological or physical. Symptoms like drug hunger often linger long after people have cleared the drug out of their system; these symptoms are endemic to all addicts and particularly intrusive for many cocaine addicts.

So, although this book focuses on cocaine addiction, it can be useful for people addicted to other drugs. It is also true that we rarely treat a person who is addicted to only one drug. There is usually at least a secondary addiction, and with cocaine addicts it is often alcohol or a downer such as Valium, which they have used to cut the edge off cocaine. Most addicts today are at least dual addicted—to two or more drugs—although often they will initially admit to only one addiction, their drug of choice, which in cases described in this book is cocaine.

Working with cocaine addicts has been challenging, frustrating, exciting, gratifying, and upsetting at various times. I have learned so much in the last few years, and I am sure I will continue to learn. My work has been rewarding, and I hope I have been able to share some of those rewards with you. I have often felt privileged to hear people's stories and to have them share so much of their lives with me. I can only hope that this book has made you a little more aware of the realities of cocaine so you are able to stay at least one step away from the line.

Appendix A

GLOSSARY

Alano Club The Alano Club is sponsored by AA and hosts various AA functions, such as meetings and dances. It provides an alternative to bars, and is a place where people who are clean and sober can meet each other.

Al-Anon Al-Anon is a fellowship of people who are affected by alcoholics and addicts. Membership consists of men and women who are friends, family, and work associates of alcoholics and addicts. The only requirement for membership is that a person feels affected by alcoholism and wants to help himself or herself and others recover from those effects. Al-Anon considers alcoholism to be a family disease and recognizes that all family members need help. There is also Nar-Anon, for people affected by narcotics abuse.

Alcoholics Anonymous (AA) "Alcoholics Anonymous is a fellowship of men and women who share their experience, strength and hope with each other that they may solve their common problem and help others to recover from alcoholism.

The only requirement for membership is a desire to stop drinking. There are no dues or fees for AA membership; we are self-supporting through our own contributions. AA is not allied with any sect, denomination, politics, organization or institution; does not wish to engage in any controversy, neither endorses nor opposes any causes. Our primary purpose is to stay sober and help alcoholics to achieve sobriety."*

---

* Permission to reprint the Preamble granted by the AA *Grapevine*.

Basers People who smoke cocaine using a method called free-basing. See *Basing*.

Basing Smoking cocaine. The cocaine is first dissolved in water, an alkali is added, and the pure cocaine is extracted with a flammable solvent, such as ether.

Blow Cocaine.

Blow it Make a mistake.

Clean Being drug free.

Clean up his act Making a change in lifestyle and eliminating drug use of any kind.

Co (also Co-dependent) A person who is close to an abuser or addict and who can and often does make it easier for the person to continue to use by covering up for him or her. A co can also learn ways of not helping a person continue to use and abuse. A co is very much affected by the addict's behavior.

Cocaine Anonymous (CA) Cocaine anonymous is a fellowship for cocaine addicts that follows the twelve step program of Alcoholics Anonymous. It is similar to AA, but geared specifically for cocaine addicts. The only requirement for membership in CA is a desire to stop using cocaine.

Cocaine high The feeling a person gets when he or she snorts, shoots, or smokes cocaine. It is initially an uplifting, euphoric feeling, but over time it becomes a dysphoric, depressive feeling.

Cocaine psychosis A reversible emotional condition precipitated by too much cocaine. Cocaine psychosis is characterized by three stages: stage one includes the following symptoms: mood swings, depression, irritability, and insomnia. Stage two symptoms are more severe than stage one, and include paranoia and anger. Stage three is characterized by rage, violence, and extreme paranoia, which may be accompanied by paranoid delusions, and auditory and visual hallucinations.

Coke Cocaine.

Connection The person a user buys cocaine from.

Cop Buy cocaine.

Crash The emotional and physical letdown after a cocaine high; also, the nervousness, irritability, and possible paranoia that can happen when the effects of cocaine wear off.

Cut A substance dealers add to cocaine in order to increase its bulk and weight (e.g., novocaine, procaine, lidocaine, speed, sugar, or talc).

Dealer A person who sells cocaine.

Dope Marijuana, heroin, or some other drug.

Down-time Some quiet, unstimulated, relaxing time to get over the cocaine high and the ensuing cocaine crash.

Edge The crash from a cocaine high. It refers to all the negative effects from the drug—both emotional and physiological.

Fire it up Lighting the freebase pipe.

Fix To shoot cocaine into a person's veins intravenously with a syringe and needle.

Freebasers See *Basers.*

Freebasing See *Basing.*

Front Give somebody cocaine on credit.

Intervention A meeting with the addict and significant others where the addict is confronted in a supportive yet confrontive way about his or her drug-taking behavior and its consequences. The intention is to get the addict to agree to enter a recovery program.

IV (intraveneous) See *Fix*.

Lines When snorting cocaine, a person usually chops the cocaine crystals into a fine powder so it can be snorted more easily, and then lays the powder out in lines so the cocaine can be snorted through a rolled-up crisp bill or straw.

Nar-Anon A fellowship of men and women that shares the AA program, but is geared towards friends and family members of narcotics abusers and addicts.

Narcotics Anonymous (NA) A fellowship of men and women that shares the AA program, but is geared towards people who have a desire to stop using narcotics.

Pinned When a person's pupils are very small as a result of using opiates, such as heroin.

Pipe A special pipe used for freebasing.

Recovery Groups Therapeutic groups for people recovering from drug addiction. They are run by counselors and therapists with experience in chemical dependency.

Reefer Marijuana.

Release of Information A form that the addict fills out so the professional involved in the addict's treatment may talk about treatment to another person; it waves certain confidentiality issues so two people may speak. The Release of Information form usually specifies what these people may talk about without denying a person's confidentiality rights.

Rig The syringe and needle used to shoot cocaine or other drugs.

Run A term used to refer to the continuous use of cocaine. The person ignores other responsibilities and focuses on getting and doing cocaine until he or she either runs out of money or passes out from exhaustion or other physiological responses to the drug (e.g., overdose).

Rush   The almost instantaneous euphoric feeling that results after a person ingests cocaine. With time, the rush can also be a surge of very negative feelings, both emotional and physical.

Score   Buy cocaine.

Shoot   Inject cocaine into a vein.

Snow   A term used to refer to cocaine.

Snort   Inhale cocaine.

Sociopaths   People with asocial or antisocial behavior or character traits. They often tell lies to make themselves look better because they think so little of themselves that they are sure if they tell the truth nobody will like them. The lies are often based on the truth, but exaggerated to make them look better.

Stash   The amount of cocaine a person has on hand for personal use.

Straight   A person who is drug-free.

Toot   The amount of cocaine a person snorts at one time.

Tracks   The small red spots left by the needles on a person's body after shooting cocaine or other drugs.

Twelve Step Program   AA, CA, NA, Al-Anon and Nar-Anon all have a twelve step program adapted from AA. A person using any of these fellowships for their recovery can utilize the outlined twelve steps to assure their continued recovery. The steps have helped millions of people stay clean and sober (see Appendix B).

White Powder Blindness   A term I use to describe a person's denial of the effects of his or her cocaine use.

Working the Steps   When people are in AA, NA, CA, or Al-Anon and are incorporating the twelve steps of that program into their daily lives, then they are working the steps. People who are actively using the steps to help them in their recovery are working the steps.

Appendix B

THE TWELVE STEPS AND TWELVE TRADITIONS

The following are the Twelve Steps and Twelve Traditions of Alcoholics Anonymous and Al-Anon. The Twelve Steps and Twelve Traditions of Narcotics Anonymous and Cocaine Anonymous are based on the Twelve Steps and Twelve Traditions of AA.

THE TWELVE STEPS OF ALCOHOLICS ANONYMOUS*

1. We admitted we were powerless over alcohol—that our lives had become unmanageable.

2. Came to believe that a Power greater than ourselves could restore us to sanity.

3. Made a decision to turn our will and our lives over to the care of God as we understood him.

4. Made a searching and fearless moral inventory of ourselves.

5. Admitted to God, to ourselves, and to another human being the exact nature of our wrongs.

6. Were entirely ready to have God remove all these defects of character.

7. Humbly asked Him to remove our shortcomings.

8. Made a list of all persons we had harmed, and became willing to make amends to them all.

9. Made direct amends to such people wherever possible, except when to do so would injure them or others.

---

* The Twelve Steps and Twelve Traditions reprinted with permission of Alcoholics Anonymous World Services, Inc.

10. Continued to take personal inventory and when we were wrong promptly admitted it.

11. Sought through prayer and meditation to improve our conscious contact with God as we understood Him, praying only for knowledge of His will for us and the power to carry that out.

12. Having had a spiritual awakening as the result of these steps, we tried to carry this message to alcoholics, and to practice these principles in all our affairs.

THE TWELVE TRADITIONS OF ALCOHOLICS ANONYMOUS (Short Form)

1. Our common welfare should come first; personal recovery depends upon AA unity.

2. For our group purpose there is but one ultimate authority— a loving God as He may express Himself in our group conscience. Our leaders are but trusted servants; they do not govern.

3. The only requirement for AA membership is a desire to stop drinking.

4. Each group should be autonomous except in matters affecting other groups or AA as a whole.

5. Each group has but one primary purpose—to carry its message to the alcoholic who still suffers.

6. An AA group ought never endorse, finance, or lend the AA name to any related facility or outside enterprise, lest problems of money, property and prestige divert us from our primary purpose.

7. Every AA group ought to be fully self-supporting, declining outside contributions.

8. Alcoholics Anonymous should remain forever nonprofessional, but our service centers may employ special workers.

9. AA, as such, ought never be organized; but we may create service boards or committees directly responsible to those they serve.

10. Alcoholics Anonymous has no opinion on outside issues; hence the AA name ought never be drawn into public controversy.

11. Our public relations policy is based on attraction rather than promotion; we need always maintain personal anonymity at the level of press, radio and films.

12. Anonymity is the spiritual foundation of all our traditions, ever reminding us to place principles before personalities.

THE TWELVE STEPS OF AL-ANON FAMILY GROUPS*

1. We admitted we were powerless over alcohol—that our lives had become unmanageable.

2. Came to believe that a power greater than ourselves could restore us to sanity.

3. Made a decision to turn our will and our lives over to the care of God *as we understood Him.*

4. Made a searching and fearless moral inventory of ourselves.

5. Admitted to God, to ourselves, and to another human being the exact nature of our wrongs.

6. Were entirely ready to have God remove all these defects of character.

7. Humbly asked Him to remove our shortcomings.

---

* From *This Is Al-Anon*, copyright 1981, by Al-Anon Family Group Headquarters, Inc. Reprinted by permission of Al-Anon Family Group Headquarters, Inc.

8. Made a list of all persons we had harmed and became willing to make amends to them all.

9. Made direct amends to such people wherever possible, except when to do so would injure them or others.

10. Continued to take personal inventory and when we were wrong, promptly admitted it.

11. Sought through prayer and meditation to improve our conscious contact with God as we understood Him, praying only for knowledge of His will for us and the power to carry that out.

12. Having had a spiritual awakening as the result of these steps, we tried to carry this message to others, and to practice these principles in all our affairs.

THE TWELVE TRADITIONS OF THE AL-ANON FAMILY GROUPS

1. Our common welfare should come first; personal progress for the greatest number depends upon unity.

2. For our group purpose there is but one authority—a loving God as He may express Himself in our group conscience. Our leaders are but trusted servants; they do not govern.

3. The relatives of alcoholics, when gathered together for mutual aid, may call themselves an Al-Anon Family Group, provided that, as a group, they have no other affiliation. The only requirement for membership is that there be a problem of alcoholism in a relative or friend.

4. Each group should be autonomous, except in matters affecting another group or Al-Anon or AA as a whole.

5. Each Al-Anon Family Group has but one purpose: to help families of alcoholics. We do this by practicing the Twelve Steps of AA *ourselves*, by encouraging and understanding our

alcoholic relatives, and by welcoming and giving comfort to families of alcoholics.

6. Our Family Groups ought never endorse, finance or lend our name to any outside enterprise, lest problems of money, property, and prestige divert us from our primary spiritual aim. Although a separate entity, we should always cooperate with Alcoholics Anonymous.

7. Every group ought to be fully self-supporting, declining outside contributions.

8. Al-Anon Twelfth-Step work should remain forever non-professional, but our service centers may employ special workers.

9. Our groups, as such, ought never be organized; but we may create service boards or committees directly responsible to those they serve.

10. The Al-Anon Family Groups have no opinion on outside issues; hence our name ought never be drawn into public controversy.

11. Our public relations policy is based on attraction rather than promotion; we need always maintain personal anonymity at the level of press, radio, films, and TV. We need guard with special care the anonymity of all AA members.

12. Anonymity is the spiritual foundation of all our traditions, ever reminding us to place principles above personalities.

References

Alcoholics Anonymous. (1976). New York: Alcoholics Anonymous World Services.

Al-Anon's Twelve Steps and Twelve Traditions. (1983). New York: Al-Anon Family Group Headquarters.

Ashley, R. (1976). *Cocaine: Its History, Uses and Effects.* New York: Warner Books.

"U.S. campaign fails to stem wave of cocaine." (February 19, 1984). *San Francisco Sunday Examiner and Chronicle,* 10.

Cohen, S. (1981). *Cocaine Today.* New York: The American Council on Marijuana and Other Psychoactive Drugs.

Gay, G. R. (1982). Clinical management of acute and chronic cocaine poisoning. *Annals of Emergency Medicine 11*(10), 562–572.

Gay, G. R. (1981). You've come a long way, baby! Coke time for the new American lady of the eighties. *Journal of Psychoactive Drugs 13*(4), 297–317.

Gold, M. S. (1984). *800-Cocaine.* Toronto: Bantam Books.

Gold, M. S. (1983). *800-Cocaine Survival Manual.* Summit, New Jersey: Fair Oaks Hospital.

Hafen, B. Q. & Frandsen, K. J. (1981). *Cocaine.* Center City, Minnesota: Hazelden.

Inaba, D. (February, 1983). *The History of Cocaine.* Presentation to Haight Ashbury Free Medical Clinic, Detoxification Project staff, San Francisco.

Magagnini, S. (August 30, 1983). Cocaine flood scares doctors. *San Francisco Chronicle*, 1, 14.

McConnell, H. (1982). Cocaine Today. *The Journal 11*,(7), 7–10.

Mortimer, G. W. (1974). *History of Coca.* San Francisco: And/Or Press.

Novey, J. H. & Zerkin, E. L. (eds.). (1982). Cocaine Smoking [Special Issue]. *Journal Of Psychoactive Drugs 14 (4).*

Petersen, R. C., Cohen, S., Jeri, F. R., Smith, D. E., and Dogoloff, L. I. (eds.). (1983). *Cocaine: A Second Look.* New York: The American Council on Marijuana and Other Psychoactive Drugs.

Phillips, J. & Wynne, R. D. (1980). *Cocaine: The Mystique and the Reality.* New York: Avon.

Seidler, G. (ed.). (1982). Cocaine [Special issue]. *Focus on Alcohol and Drug Issues 5(4).*

Stern, B. (Producer), Chilnick, L. D. (ed.), Garrett, R. C., Waldmeyer, U. G., and Sernaque, V. (Text), Smith, D. E., and Seymour, R. B. (Medical Consultants). (1984). *The Coke Book.* New York: Berkley Books.

Twelve Steps and Twelve Traditions. (1974). New York: Alcoholics Anonymous World Services.